STONED

The Truth About Medical Marijuana and Hemp Oil

James W. Forsythe, M.D., H.M.D.

Pat & Bob
Stay "high" on
life itself!
James W Forsythe MD, HMD

Stoned ~ The Truth About Medical Marijuana and Hemp Oil
Century Wellness Publishing

Copyright (c) 2015, By James W. Forsythe, M.D., H.M.D.
All Rights Reserved, including the right of reproduction in
whole or in part in any form.

Forsythe, James W M.D., H.M.D.
1. Health 2. Homeopathy 3. Cancer
Book Design: Patty Atcheson Melton

ISBN:978-0-9897636-5-3

Dedication

To all patients who use hemp oil in a successful desire to obtain a long-term remission of their Stage IV cancers ... and, to Bret Bocook, who suffered from two separate brain cancers. Bocook became a natural-treatment pioneer, living more than five years thanks to hemp oil-maintenance therapy. I consider him a major trailblazer for future patients.

To my "California connection," Constance Finley, a remarkable scientist who single-handedly developed a milestone hemp oil formula. Her creation has produced a prolonged remission rate of more than 90 percent, among a small group (28) of Stage IV adult cancer patients. This serves as significant evidence of hemp oil's great value as a tremendous asset in maintenance therapy.

Also, a special thanks to my research editor, Wayne Rollan Melton, and graphic designer and artist Patty Atcheson-Melton, for their extraordinary work in the preparation of this book.

Editor's Note

Please note that for simplicity purposes, whenever the word "cannabis" is used that term usually indicates either or both primary strains of the plant--marijuana and hemp.

Contents

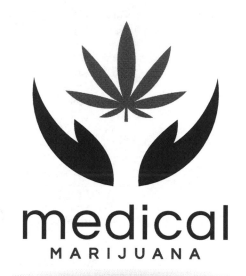

medical
MARIJUANA

1
The Medicinal Marijuana Craze

A relentless tidal wave of popularity has sharply increased the widespread use of marijuana for medicinal purposes across the United States.

Yet rampant misinformation has clouded the issue, as many people use bogus or fraudulent claims regarding their personal health as a fake excuse to use the drug.

Worsening matters, streams of people who actually might benefit from cannabis fail to effectively administer the substance in a manner likely help them.

The concern intensifies even more when taking into account the fact that the federal government classifies marijuana as illegal. People convicted in federal courts of using, possessing, cultivating and selling cannabis face mandatory prison time.

The proverbial waters get rippled even more when taking into account the fact that each U.S. territory and state has its own unique marijuana laws. These factors heighten the overall confusion; some jurisdictions classify this natural substance as "legal for recreational use," while other governments list possession as a felony.

People Asked Me for Help
Amid the resulting media hubbub, streams of news stories in recent years have hailed marijuana as a "wonder drug" for curing many diseases--particularly cancer.

Motivated to discover the "truth" and craving a source of accurate information, people from around the world have asked me to write this book.

You see, many doctors and patients from around the globe

consider me one of the world's premiere cancer treatment experts.

Much of the interest stems from the fact that my clinic in Reno, Nevada, has one of the world's greatest success rates at treating the worse cancers.

This becomes possible because I'm an extremely rare type of physician; as an integrative medical oncologist I'm licensed to administer mainstream drugs including chemotherapy--and also natural, effective and safe homeopathic remedies.

The five-year remission or "cure" rate of advanced Stage IV cancer patients at my Century Wellness Clinic is far better than obtained by mainstream doctors.

Only two out of every 100 such patients remain alive after five years when treated nationwide by conventional physicians. This compares with an average 65 survivors out of every 100 similar patients treated at my clinic.

People Seek my Professional Advice

Now in my fifth decade as a practicing oncologist, I have written or been mentioned positively in more than 20 books on important medical issues.

Among the most popular was the runaway 2010 bestseller by media personality Suzanne Somers, "Knockout: Interviews with Doctors who are Curing Cancer."

Heralding me as a "Renaissance man" in the area of cancer treatment, Somers said my qualifications make for an "interesting mix of Western and alternative medicines.

"The combination of the two allows Doctor Forsythe to be extremely creative in his approach to cancer"--providing, in his words, 'the best of what both worlds have to offer.' Today, Doctor Forsythe enjoys a successful career as a medical oncologist who utilizes alternative treatments, and patients flock to him from all over the world for his cutting-edge treatments."

The overall patient totals at my clinic continue to steadily increase, thanks largely to the fact that people worldwide yearn for effective natural remedies. On any given week, my clinic's parking lot hosts vehicles from as far away as Maine, Florida and Alaska. Century Wellness Clinic has regularly treated patients from every continent except Antarctica.

A "Perfect Storm" Erupted

An increase in the popularity of marijuana as a "remedy," coupled with my expertise, has generated a "perfect storm" that resulted in this book's publication.

The Internet is crammed with misinformation involving this critical issue, riddled with enough holes to resemble an aged block of Swiss cheese.

The overall challenge becomes even more formidable when taking into account the fact that most books about medicinal marijuana have misleading data. Only a handful were written by medical doctors, those best qualified to analyze this unique issue.

"Consumers who embrace virtually everything they're told about the 'Miracle of Weed,' risk breaking the law--while endangering their own health," I sometimes tell patients eager to learn more. "Avoid such trouble by listening to reputable sources."

Unlike the majority of so-called 'Pot Experts,' as a physician I have carefully studied and analyzed this issue for many years. My Number One priority always focuses on the optimal health and general welfare of patients, wanting the best for them and for their families.

Although medicinal marijuana products including "cannabis oil" are not available through my clinic, I'm a certified medical expert on effective natural remedies that mainstream physicians choose to ignore or discount.

Medicinal Marijuana Works Wonders

From the start here, I'm delighted to report that when used properly under a trained physician's careful guidance, medicinal marijuana often "works wonders" in addressing a wide variety of serious ailments--particularly cancer.

Consumers who fail to follow sound medical advice and criteria invariably put their own health at great risk. When administered in a haphazard fashion without a well-laid-out action plan and the guidance of a medical professional, most self-administered health-maintenance regimens invariably fail.

Trying to cure your own cancer without following a solid action plan is the equivalent of attempting to fly a jet aircraft without first getting extensive lessons. People who jump into the pilot's seat without the benefit of training invariably end in disaster.

A significant question should emerge for current and prospective "weed patients" yearning to achieve good health: "Am I only doing this as an excuse to get high, or more important, have I chosen the best strategies for using pot to cure my ailment?"

After deep reflection on such queries, some consumers admit that they merely want to enjoy the euphoric sensations made possible by marijuana. For them, using the "playing card of health" to get high becomes a high-risk game.

Consider Your Personal Situation

Before launching a health-enhancement effort with marijuana, anyone serious about getting positive results should first carefully study the essential information that I have provided in the pages that follow.

This way from the start you will know all the essential basics necessary to understand the many potential benefits on your pathway to possibly getting "cured."

With equal importance, you also can learn of the numerous pitfalls likely to impose formidable danger. Many so-called medical marijuana experts refrain from acknowledging that such proverbial landmines even exist.

As you're about to discover, many possible problems emerge,

not the least of which is becoming a pothead or a person that much of society categorizes as a "loser."

Even among those who "could not care less what other people think," everyone embarking on such a journey must acknowledge that there is a "right way and a wrong way" for administering medicinal marijuana.

This is No Joking Matter

Your personal and mental health are far from a "joking matter."

Think of the situation this way. If behaving like most people, you would never buy an expensive, top-of-the-line house only to smash it with a wrecking ball.

Well, without exaggeration, your body and mind are the equivalent of your own home--virtually essential, the start-point and end-point for everything in your life.

Yes, your body and mind are the "essence of you" that we're talking about. So, avoid obliterating your precious mind and your unique, blessed body. This means avoiding reckless behavior likely to endanger your long-term health.

When administered the "right way," marijuana can restore good health or at the very least effectively and safely mask the negative signs of adverse symptoms. Conversely, the reckless and rampant use of cannabis without a positive action plan might irreparably damage your mind and body.

My Task Becomes Crystal Clear

Now that I have clearly established basics of this proverbial playing field you will soon discover the many risks and rewards involved.

Mapping out and explaining the most essential of these details becomes fairly easy. All you'll need to do is understand the basics before following a step-by-step action plan.

In order to excel at any sport, artistic endeavor, family life and business, a clear understanding and continual review of the basics serves as a necessary starting point.

The selection, dosages and administering techniques involving psychoactive cannabis hail as as equally important processes. With this criteria established as a necessary foundation, here are the basics of what you soon will learn much more about:

The Product: What is marijuana, and what does it do within the body to generate psychoactive effects--the mental sensations of euphoria--the famous "high?"

Marijuana Receptors: What are the receptors or biological characteristics within marijuana that enable this natural substance to naturally interact with the body?

Cancer Receptors: What are the biological receptors within cancer that accept the marijuana chemicals, a process that often "kills the disease?"

Hemp Oil: Why and how is hemp oil, actually made from a non-hemp subspecies of marijuana, by far the most preferred and most effective marijuana-based substance that naturally destroys cancer?

Making Cannabis Oil: Learn how the most effective and highly concentrated "hemp oil" is produced, plus where and how to obtain this substance. Although often called hemp oil, this substance actually comes from cannabis strains that lack the primary attributes of hemp--sometimes used for industrial purposes.

Using "Cannabis Oil": Learn the best ways to administer the oil, plus the necessary quantities and timetables for eradicating cancer.

Learn Psychoactive Attributes: Learn why at least some psychoactive qualities are required in order for hemp oil to effectively eradicate cancer.

Certified Doctors: Learn why and how you need to find licensed, certified doctors to guide and monitor your medicinal use of marijuana or hemp oil.

Address Ailments: Besides cancer, what are the numerous

ailments that marijuana can "cure" or alleviate, and how does this happen?

Snake Oil: How--if at all--are marijuana and hemp like a "snake oil," a supposed Miracle Drug or cure-all for virtually every physical affliction known to mankind?

Positive Results: What are the specific potential positive results of using cannabis or hemp oil for medicinal purposes?

Negative Results: What are some of the potential negative physical outcomes from the long-term or even short-term use of this natural substance.

Illegal Substance: Why you should always remain fully cognizant that marijuana is listed as illegal in many jurisdictions, which have widely varying criminal penalties.

Money Matters: How much will the marijuana or hemp products cost, particularly for the effective amounts needed to eradicate your cancer or other diseases?

Boundless Possibilities Emerge

Upon learning the benefits and uses of "Miraculous Marijuana" and "Happy Hemp," consumers can easily put themselves on track for potentially huge benefits.

All along, each person needs to remain cognizant of the supreme need to comply with all local, state and national laws that vary significantly worldwide.

All consumers and even recreational users of marijuana have a personal responsibility to know and to comply with such regulations. As a result, this book never advocates or condones the illicit use of this natural and generally harmless substance.

Just like water and even oxygen, all natural substances including marijuana can emerge as extremely harmful or even deadly when used in extremely large amounts.

New and even current users of psychoactive cannabis also need to remain fully cognizant of the fact that driving while "high" on marijuana can cause serious accidents. Adding to the woes of such users, criminal convictions in such instances often lead to lengthy prison sentences.

Benefits Outweigh the Negatives

People who manage to legally use marijuana for medicinal purposes, as allowed in certain jurisdictions, often experience a far greater number of physical and psychological benefits--as opposed to the limited number so-called "negatives."

Ultimately, the possession and use of marijuana for medical purposes often becomes a personal decision. Just as no one should ever be forced to consume alcohol, society should never require people to use marijuana.

Even so, consumers and patients everywhere should have a right to learn and to benefit from the many proven medical benefits that this leafy green substance provides.

Although marijuana laws have recently loosed up somewhat in certain jurisdictions worldwide, much of society still portrays this natural substance as "evil."

Sure enough, marijuana and even hemp have been labeled by some law enforcement experts as "gateway drugs," supposedly leading to the use of much more dangerous and often-deadly narcotics such as meth, heroin, LSD and morphine.

Yet rather than portray marijuana in such 100-percent negative terms, government leaders and doctors need to "open up about the issue." Officials and experts can and should acknowledge the many fantastic potential health benefits, particularly in the treatment, potential eradication and control of cancer.

The Gateway to Improved Health

Rather than incorrectly labeling hemp and marijuana as a "gateway to illicit narcotics," health professionals worldwide need to do a much better job at accurately and honestly portraying these substances as a "phenomenal doorway to better health."

As a doctor highly experienced at "curing" or controlling

cancer, I have a personal responsibility to inform the world about these stupendous details.

Throughout history many of the world's greatest philosophers, religious leaders and even scientists have proclaimed that "the truth will set you free."

The simple and irrefutable fact here, as fully chronicled in the pages that follow, is that the marijuana oil--sometimes called "hemp oil" or "weed oil"--can powerfully control cancer when correctly administered.

Sadly, however, the vast majority of mainstream doctors and oncologists invariably frown at the very mention of such claims. They describe such supposedly "bogus medicine" as "pure quackery." Some physicians claim that far more comprehensive studies are needed to provide any possible proof. Until that happens, they say, "outlaw marijuana and impose much more stringent restrictions on its medicinal use."

Yet the many positive facts that follow in this publication leave little or no room for doubt, because when used properly, psychoactive cannabis serves as an essential and vital ally in effectively controlling disease and severe physical afflictions. Once consumers learn these essential details, authorities will find themselves unable to deny the truth.

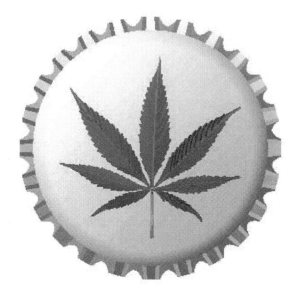

2
Marijuana
The Basic Details

Before learning highly detailed specifics about medicinal marijuana, consumers must know the basic side effects and also the potential dangers.

Remember, as previously stated, using marijuana is generally safe for the vast majority of adults when used at moderate levels, well below the "certified stoner" range.

With this understood, consumers also need to realize that many people claim scientists still lack a full understanding of marijuana's long-term effects.

Despite such concerns, a vast majority of long-term cannabis users claim that when used for many years, the drug fails to generate adverse side effects.

Cognizant of these conflicting opinions, any person who decides to use this natural substance needs to know that doing so "is done at your own risk."

Thus, before trying "weed" for the first time, or even for long-time users, learning the side effects and basic attributes becomes essential.

Primary Purposes

Some of the following answers and explanations might seem obvious, but they are good to know. Lots of marijuana users-- including those who have used the drug for many years--express shock, dismay or even a sense of delight when learning these details.

Atop the list of basics here are some primary yet essential details, much of which many people already know about. Yet the details are worth repeating here, especially before additional, extensive follow-up information in subsequent chapters.

Just about everyone knows the general uses of marijuana, but both attributes need a brief mention here--because each will receive extensive explanation later in this book:

Getting high: Whether society as a whole admits this or not, an increasingly large percentage of the U.S. population that uses cannabis does so merely to "get high."

Medicinal reasons: Many people insist that marijuana serves as the only reliable, relatively safe substance in addressing their personal health issues.

Moral Issues Enter the Fray

The moral issue of whether marijuana is "good or evil" has become particularly prevalent throughout much of American society.

Largely for these reasons, in the pages that follow you'll learn about the drug's history, plus the evolution of laws on marijuana prohibitions or distribution.

Along the way, you'll discover why many people detest marijuana on moral or religious grounds, often although they have never tried this substance.

Just as important, consumers need to know how and why marijuana regulations were imposed--plus details on the current trend of loosening or eliminating these laws.

Once these interworking details become clear to them, many people admit that they're amazed to learn these undeniably fascinating details.

Awe-Inspiring Information

With great certainty, I can predict with confidence that by the time they reach the final page the vast majority of readers likely will find details that leave them somewhat mystified or even filled with awe.

Along this journey, you'll learn how marijuana and its related plant, hemp, have generated a significant impact on hundreds of diverse cultures worldwide.

Additional intrigue often emerges upon learning of the many ways to smoke, eat or use marijuana--plus the psychoactive experience people have when getting high.

For instance, did you know that there are many types of "high" from cannabis. These attributes range from a sense of euphoria and enhanced humor, to a rapid acceleration in creativity and risk-taking--all hinged on the specific strain of plant.

Even more curiosity peaks upon discovering the many unique comparisons between marijuana and a vast array of other drugs, particularly alcohol.

Just as essential, how, why and where is most marijuana sold to U.S. consumers grown and produced? Why and how have specific new cannabis strains been developed since the start of the 21st Century? Compared to the 1990s, why and how have today's average potencies increased for typical marijuana products available for medical and recreational use? And what has caused the recent surge in consumer demand?

The Proverbial Train Keeps Moving

Whether authorities care to admit this or not, a proverbial freight train that signifies America's use of this drug keeps moving at an increasingly fast rate.

If the recent strides in loosening marijuana laws is any indication, growing numbers of consumers are likely to demand more of the drug--especially strains or crops considered highly potent.

Ironically, these rapid-fire transitions impact all of U.S. society just as advances in cannabis farming technology accelerates total nationwide marijuana production and sales.

For these reasons, you'll also learn the latest cannabis growing techniques used by many of the world's most proficient and productive marijuana growers.

In the process, readers also will discover the "right" and "wrong" ways that marijuana is grown, in some instances recklessly endangering consumer health.

Unique Consumption Methods

Besides discovering the many unique and diverse ways of smoking marijuana, you'll also learn of numerous ways to bake or cook the plant for eating.

Many ill-informed people, most who have never tried psychoactive cannabis, have never realized that eating marijuana can generate a stupendous high.

So, how, when and why are marijuana foods prepared? Just as essential from the standpoint of people who like to get stoned, which is best--food or smoking?

Another essential factor to consider becomes medicinal. For those who insist that they need marijuana for medical reasons, which consumption method generates ideal health benefits--smoking, eating or a combination of both?

Also, from the viewpoint of general consumers who simply want to get high, how much marijuana is considered too much for health reasons? Additionally, how many people have died from marijuana overdoses--and how does this occur, if ever?

Everyone Needs to Know

Virtually every adult nationwide needs to know the many essential details regarding marijuana.

A primary reason stems from the undeniable fact that psychoactive cannabis rapidly seems to be growing so fast in popularity that the drug is becoming as pervasive as alcohol across America--at least from the view of some observers.

Cognizant of these changes, people, families and organizations that have been "on the sidelines" on these issues until now can no longer ignore the problems.

Law enforcement officials, drug rehabilitation experts and

public research polls indicate that in recent decades virtually all American families have been impacted by illicit drugs including marijuana.

If public surveys are an accurate indication, then cannabis reigns as by far the most popular illicit drug in the nation-- although as previously stated the growth, possession, use and sale of marijuana remains a felony under federal law.

For these reasons, everyone today has a responsibility to learn about psychoactive cannabis, everything from potential dangers to apparent benefits.

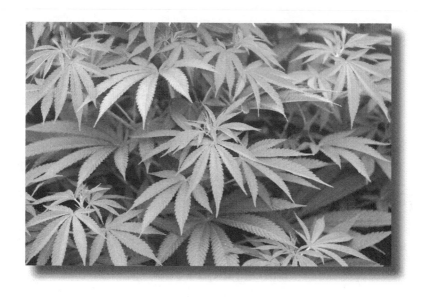

3
Marijuana and Hemp 101: Discover the Basics

Varying public surveys and polls have estimated that anywhere from 5 percent to 25 percent of Americans have tried marijuana at least once.

Annual surveys in recent years have indicated that the percentage of U.S. citizens who regularly use the substance has steadily increased without signs of letup.

Indeed, overall public acceptance has remained on the rise, particularly as more people learn about marijuana's many positive benefits.

By some accounts, for the first time in history in recent years more than half of people surveyed in public opinion polls indicated that they approve of medical marijuana.

Even so, the vast majority of people lack any inkling of how marijuana works, at least based on my personal experience and stories posted in the mainstream media.

Perhaps just as disturbing, many politicians still insist on imposing overly harsh anti-marijuana laws. Equally distressing, the mainstream drug industry--sometimes called "Big Pharma"-- also strives to portray cannabis in a negative light.

The multi-billion dollar pharmaceutical industry stands to lose huge income, perhaps many billions of dollars, if and when marijuana is fully legalized.

Instead of buying expensive, dangerous and addictive drugs made by Big Pharma, if and when psychoactive cannabis is fully legalized consumers would be able to purchase or grow marijuana or medicinal hemp.

Such an outcome would enrage Big Pharma because by law pharmaceutical companies are prohibited from obtaining patents on natural substances. "Made by Mother Nature" products include plants found growing in the wild, including cannabis.

Big Pharma Builds Roadblock

Determined to protect "its own best-interests," Big Pharma has played an integral role in getting politicians to impose and maintain harsh anti-cannabis laws.

Many people remain unaware of the disturbing fact that Big Pharma and the alcohol industry each have many thousands of high-paid lobbyists.

These professionals have expertise at strong-arming and manipulating politicians who work in state capitols nationwide and in Washington, D.C., the hub of the U.S. government.

The majority of lawmakers invariably cave in to the urgings of these lobbyists, partly due to huge campaign donations doled out by the drug industry.

Compounding this problem multi-fold, the various federal government agencies involved in health issues are loaded with Big Pharma allies.

These include doctors and scientists, most who attended medical schools and universities that all have close ties to the pharmaceutical industry. The vast majority of these students are taught that "unnatural, synthetic drugs are the only way to go"--while any unnatural substances including vitamins, herbs and plants are nothing but "quackery."

Consumers Seize Control of the Issue

Thankfully, consumers in a limited number of states have legally seized at least some control of the issue in recent years via the right to vote.

Voters in Washington state and Colorado helped lead the way by deciding to legalize separate types of recreational marijuana laws in their states.

Just as important, in recent decades consumers in numerous

other states have convinced their legislators to approve medical marijuana laws within those jurisdictions.

Sadly, in many instances during the past few decades this proverbial whirlwind of rapid change has resulted in a virtual "Pot-Gone-Wild" situation where far too many medical marijuana stores operated in some communities.

In some instances these problems worsened when consumers received bogus marijuana prescriptions from people parading as so-called medical experts; in far too many instances, these crooks are actually individuals with nefarious backgrounds. Such charlatans lack scientific or medical experience.

These negative factors in turn motivated some communities such as those in Los Angeles to shut down, ban or highly regulate what previously had been the rampant saturation of medical marijuana dispensaries.

Feds Muddy the Issue

While the proverbial whirlpool of conflicting or diverse local and state laws continued swirling non-stop, the federal government has muddied the issue to the detriment of consumers nationwide.

As previously indicated, the federal government continues to list the possession, use, growth and distribution of cannabis as a top-class felony.

People convicted of such offenses in federal court face mandatory prison time and extensive fines, much to the delight of Big Pharma and the alcohol industry. Both want to block and punish such competitors.

Some people fully aware of this disturbing situation might in turn want to classify the federal government as corrupt, a crony that kowtows to big business, lobbyists, and particularly Big Pharma.

Lacking the legal power to curtail these lawmakers and bureaucrats, some consumers who yearn for the health benefits of cannabis feel as if "stuck in the middle."

Controversies erupted as "budding entrepreneurs" created and operated extensive marijuana-growing and distribution facilities in states that have legalized the drug.

Yet many of these business operators learned the hard way that the federal government plays no favorites when carrying out the wishes of Big Pharma and major alcohol manufacturing companies.

On a sporadic and scattered basis, even within states that have legalized medical marijuana, "the feds" have arrested and convicted operators of such major businesses. Many offenders were slapped with minimum ten-year prison sentences, capped off with monetary fines reaching hundreds of thousands of dollars in some instances.

Overabundance of Pot

Authorities have learned the hard way that extensive problems occur, even in some jurisdictions where voters have legalized marijuana for recreational use. Among some of the most disturbing, significant or difficult-to-manage challenges:

Excessive production: Eager to maximize revenues, some licensed sellers of marijuana in Washington state grew far too much cannabis. The occasional overabundance of pot sometimes resulted in instances where storage facilities were crammed with the substance. The entrepreneurs in these instances lacked enough consumers to purchase the product.

Business security: Due largely to the massive quantities of cash and valuable cannabis products, licensed dispensaries in Washington state, Colorado, Oregon, Alaska, and the District of Colombia have had to employ extensive armed security forces. These are necessary to thwart thieves including organized criminals eager to steal vaults of cash and truckloads of pot to sell elsewhere.

Monetary problems: Psychoactive cannabis vendors in Washington state and Colorado, plus medical marijuana dispensaries nationwide, refuse to accept credit cards or even bank-issued debit cards. This refusal stems from the fact that financial institutions--including credit card companies--face the revocation of their required federal licenses, if and when processing funds from the production and sale of marijuana. As a result, legalized marijuana dispensaries operate as cash-only businesses.

Misinformation: Authorities and licensed sellers have learned the hard way that many consumers lack the essential and critical knowledge of how much cannabis they can safely consume and when. A primary example here involved a journalist from the East Coast who ate an entire marijuana-laced candy bar in Colorado in a brief single session--rather than ingesting the treat in small quantities in intervals over an extended period of time. The woman reported that she unwittingly got severely stoned, to the point that she became became bedridden and unable to function for many hours. Partly as a result, the licensed-marijuana sales businesses have tried to implement accurate product labeling and public education.

Difficult Issues Will Remain

The use, possession and distribution of marijuana and "weed oil" are likely to remain challenging and controversial issues throughout the 21st Century, and perhaps for hundreds of years to come.

The probability of a universal, comprehensive and widely accepted cannabis law seems low, due to the complexity and the supposed morality of the many controversial factors involved.

The overall issue will remain divisive, at least in some ways like the continually heated and never-ending abortion controversy. Of course, these separate and unrelated challenges lack any direct connection.

Yet these overall non-stop debates share distinct similarities. The anti-abortion and pro-abortion advocates each claim to hold the highest "moral ground," while supposedly backed by their separate, conflicting versions of "reliable science." Each group refuses to change or even slightly modify its political position.

With little doubt the pro-weed and anti-weed advocates also each seem to claim that God or Mother Nature are "on our side." The anti-cannabis crowd contends the substance injures the body and mind, while adversaries argue the opposite.

Jump Off the Proverbial Treadmill

Those with extreme positions on each contrasting side of the marijuana issue behave as if mice stuck on a non-stop treadmill while locked in cages.

On an overall societal scale, the cannabis debate mirrors what everyday citizens see regularly throughout most of American society.

With increased frequency since the 21st Century began, sociologists have contended that American society is virtually being "split down the middle" on key issues.

Controversies sparking heated arguments and protests have ranged from abortion and race relations to politics, cannabis, health care and much more.

All these intense debates are important to mention at least briefly during any comprehensive discussion regarding the future of how society uses and regulates medical and recreational marijuana.

Ultimately, each side of the cannabis debate accuses the other of "junk science." Naturally as a result, the Internet is crammed with a wide range of diverse claims that cannabis dramatically improves health--while just as many statements contend otherwise.

Cut to the Chase

As previously stated, while determined to slice through mounds of misinformation and get at the "truth," I have spent many years scouring through scientific documentation regarding cannabis.

My findings are likely to shock and even anger the anti-marijuana crowd.

You see, as previously indicated, irrefutable evidence exists to substantiate the claim that when used "the right way" under proper medical guidance cannabis alleviates many physical ailments.

Perhaps most important of all in this regard, oil from cannabis often eradicates the most deadly cancers.

Despite these miraculous medicinal qualities, however, any reports regarding my findings here are likely to do little if anything to sway opinions of the anti-cannabis crowd.

As with all of today's significant controversies, the marijuana issue has drawn proponents and opponents who choose to take a close-minded approach. No amount of verifiable information regarding the positive effects of cannabis will prompt many anti-marijuana advocates to change the minds.

Even so, the public deserves and has a right to the essential and positive information that I have provided here--particularly regarding the control of cancer.

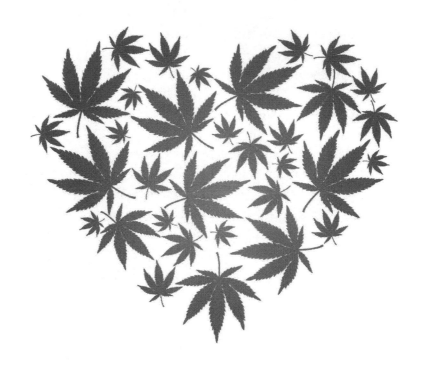

4
Positive Comments About Marijuana Intensify

With increasing frequency in recent years, average people including celebrities nationwide have made strong but positive comments supporting marijuana.

One of the most famous of these statements came from Sanjay Gupta, an internationally acclaimed neurosurgeon and assistant professor of neurology.

In 2013, Gupta famously changed his mind about cannabis, two years after writing an article for "Time" magazine entitled "Why I would vote no on pot."

Gupta admitted that when forming his initial opinion, he had scoured government documentation regarding marijuana, "but I didn't look hard enough."

Later, however, while developing a documentary for CNN entitled "Weed," Gupta interviewed patients and medical experts worldwide about the drug.

"I apologize because I didn't look hard enough until now," Gupta said, his updated comments still available for review on the international news network's Website. "I didn't look hard enough; I didn't review papers from smaller labs in other countries doing some remarkable research, and I was too submissive of the loud chorus of legitimate patients whose symptoms improved on cannabis."

Courageous Reversal of Opinion

In changing his mind about the drug, Gupta showed the kind of wisdom, courage and fortitude that many mainstream doctors are unwilling to make.

Far too many of today's physicians take a timid, wait-and-see stance; these doctors steer away from recommending the drug while repetitively proclaiming "more research needs to be done."

Today's fast-paced society needs many more mainstream physicians of Gupta's respected status to drop their opposition to effective natural remedies such as marijuana.

By the time he reversed his opinion Gupta even had enough spunk to admit that regarding people who advocate medicinal cannabis "I lumped them with the high-visibility maligners, just looking to get high.

"I mistakenly believed the U.S. Drug Enforcement Agency (Administration) listed marijuana as a Schedule I substance because of sound scientific proof. Surely they must have quality reasoning as to why marijuana is in the category of the most dangerous drugs that have 'no accepted medical use and a high potential for abuse.'"

Yet upon reversing his opinion, however, Gupta concluded that the federal government lacks scientific evidence to back its claim.

Accentuating the Positives

When researching and filming "Weed," Gupta met lots of patients whose health improved substantially as a result of using medicinal marijuana.

Perhaps the most famous of these patients is Charlotte Figi, who began suffering up to 300 daily life-threatening and dangerous seizures caused by "Dravet" Syndrome, a severe myoclonic epilepsy. Charlotte's doctors initially tried seven different mainstream Big Pharma anti-convulsant drugs that each failed to relieve her debilitating symptoms.

As a last course, the physicians began giving the girl medicinal marijuana, which almost immediately relieved symptoms. With her brain finally calmed, two years after her cannabis treatments began the girl suffered only two or three seizures monthly, according to numerous news reports.

Encouraged by a steadily growing number of similarly positive results, patients advocating medicinal marijuana and some doctors are working more than ever in efforts to legalize medical cannabis.

Bravely when announcing his position reversal, Gupta wrote that "We have been terribly and systematically misled for nearly 70 years in the United States, and I apologize for my role in that."

Positive Attitude Spreads

Energized by statements such as those by Gupta, many average people are using the Internet to publicly proclaim their support for medicinal marijuana.

Some of these individuals include entire families featured in videos shown on YouTube, everyone weeping for joy after marijuana oil "cured" them or their relatives.

At least according to those featured in the videos, the patients previously had been informed by mainstream doctors to "get your affairs in order. You only have a few months left until you run out of time."

Tragically, despite such intense and positive proclamations, mainstream physicians and the American Medical Association ignore statements such as these, always repetitively proclaiming that much more study is needed.

As if adding insult to injury, mainstream physicians have never bothered to study the medicinal effects of marijuana on a massive and unbiased scale.

Despite this ongoing setback, although marijuana remains illegal under federal law, many people nationwide remain busy spreading ballot initiatives; these would let voters decide on whether to legalize marijuana and matters involving medical cannabis.

Federal Government Lacked Documented Studies

In reversing his opinion on marijuana, Gupta revealed that he had discovered what he called an "unsettling" 1970 statement from a top federal government health official. The controversial comment had been made by then-Assistant Secretary of Health, Doctor Roger O. Egeberg, when recommending that the plant be classified under Schedule I:

"Since there is still a considerable void in our knowledge of the plant and effects of the active drug in it, our recommendation is that marijuana be retained within Schedule I--at least until the completion of certain studies now underway to resolve the issue."

Gupta discovered to his disappointment that those studies never were completed, and that Egeberg ignored research from the mid-1940s, which concluded that using marijuana generally fails to generate serious consequences.

At least one of those reports was commissioned in 1944 by the then-New York City Mayor Fiorello LaGuardia; that research concluded that cannabis never causes serious addiction. That study also failed to find evidence that the plant leads to addictions of dangerous drugs like heroin, morphine and cocaine.

Gupta said that although marijuana sometimes leads to withdrawal symptoms like anxiety, nausea and insomnia, "it is hard to make a case that it has a high potential for abuse." He also said that despite the general overall safety of marijuana, "developing brains are likely more susceptible to harm than adult brains."

Charlotte Created a Sensation

Gupta's initial and follow-up reports on Charlotte Figi created somewhat of a media sensation, generating intense nationwide demand for the strain of marijuana used to treat her and named in her honor--Charlotte's Web.

That strain of marijuana originally had been called "Hippie's Disappointment" because it contains an extremely small percentage of THC, according to a 2013 report by the CBS Television affiliate in Denver.

Most popular cannabis strains that generate what users describe as a fantastic high usually have a THC content from 15 percent to

25 percent. From the perspective of many marijuana users, "the higher percentage of THC, the better--by far."

By contrast, Charlotte's Web plants have THC contents of much lower than a mere 1 percent.

Rather than "smoking weed," the little girl eats an olive oil solution that contains a high concentration of non-psychoactive cannabinoid substances from the plant named in her honor. The extract is either placed on her tongue or in her food, according to various news media reports.

Sensational Demand Surges

Streams of separate news reports individually and collectively indicated that demand for Charlotte's Web skyrocketed nationwide following the broadcasts of Gupta's initial documentary on the issue, "Weed," and his follow-up film, "Weed 2."

More than 12,000 families were placed on a waiting list for the drug, desperate to find remedies after standard Big Pharma pharmaceuticals failed to block seizures in their children suffering from epilepsy, according to a 2014 report in "Time" magazine.

The "New York Times" had already reported in December 2013 that families eager to get these remedies for their children "flocked" to Colorado after that state legalized recreational marijuana.

Demand intensified so much that in November 2013 Denver's CBS-TV affiliate said that 93 families with epileptic children were already using marijuana daily, while "hundreds are on the waiting list, and thousands are calling."

The issue received additional traction in the news media when journalists labeled the streams of families migrating to Colorado as "medicinal marijuana refugees," forced to leave states that prohibit medical cannabis.

Caution and More Research Urged

The demand for medicinal marijuana and public awareness of the drug's many benefits have outpaced old, tired and senseless government policy on the issue.

This dilemma has been called a "Catch-22" situation, largely because far more research is needed. As previously stated, the production, use, possession and sale of marijuana remains classified under Schedule I of federal law, a high-level felony.

Gupta discovered when researching for "Weed" that only one marijuana farm is authorized to produce the plant for scientific research, located in Mississippi on the Ole Miss campus. Announcing his changed opinion on the marijuana issue, Gupta said when he visited the campus in 2013 "there was no marijuana being grown."

Further complicating matters, the process of researching marijuana and then getting the findings reviewed becomes "tedious" for several reasons. Among them:

Cancer: Any report must be reviewed and eventually approved by the National Cancer Institute.

Pain: Any findings or research on how cannabis relieves pain likely would have to be reviewed by the National Institute for Neurological Disorders.

Required approvals: The National Institute on Drug Abuse likely would have to review the research. Yet Gupta describes that institution as "an organization that has a core mission of studying drug abuse, as opposed to benefit."

Legitimate Patients Suffer

Sadly, legitimate patients who need medicinal marijuana end up squeezed out of the process in this senseless, cumbersome and tragic bureaucratic maze.

Through a personal "trial-and-error process" lots of these individuals have discovered that marijuana works by far the best for them. This usually happens without generating the many negative side effects and without the dangers of standard drugs.

Even more confusion and disappointment emerges from the fact that the medical marijuana laws created by most states have sparked a hodgepodge of confusion. Each state that permits medicinal cannabis has its own unique laws regulating this process--banning some health-related uses while allowing others.

As a prime example, Colorado permits medicinal cannabis to treat eight conditions ranging from seizures and severe pain to addressing weight loss, cancer and glaucoma. Other states that permit medical marijuana have vastly different rules.

Further complicating these matters, elected officials who lack any medical educations and who have no well-informed knowledge on the issue are making these so-called "life-and-death decisions."

"Dreams" verses "Nightmares"

The various issues already mentioned have collectively been hailed as "a scientist's dream and a doctor's nightmare."

According to a maze of news reports lots of physicians have expressed both concern and worry. These conflicting and sometimes confusing opinions have suddenly clicked into full gear in recent years, while overall public demand for medical marijuana surges--much faster than that rate of new reliable research into cannabis.

A 2013 article in "The Oklahoman" helped put this confusing dilemma into perspective, quoting Charlotte Figi's physician, Alan Shakelford, as admitting: "We really don't know how it works. The cannabidiol seems to act as a neuro-stabilizer, but how? The research is minuscule on this."

Par for the course, despite the obvious effectiveness of marijuana in treating some epileptic patients, the American Epilepsy Society has seemed to downplay or perhaps even side-step the obvious positive medical attributes of cannabis.

In early 2014 the Society said that "while there are some anecdotal reports of marijuana use in treating epilepsy, scientific evidence for the routine use of marijuana for this indication is lacking. The lack of information does not mean that marijuana is ineffective for epilepsy. It merely means that we do not know if marijuana is a safe and efficacious treatment for epilepsy.

"In addition, little is known about the long-term effects of using marijuana in infants and children, and chronic exposure during adolescence has been shown to have lasting negative effects on cognition and mood. Such safety concerns coupled with a lack of evidence of efficacy in controlled studies result in a risk-benefit ratio that does not support (the) use of marijuana for treatment of seizures at this time."

Mind-Boggling Conclusions

Statements such as those by the American Epilepsy Society are "nothing short of mind-boggling" to some users of medicinal marijuana.

For the most part standard medications typically prescribed by mainstream physicians for treating epilepsy have been known to cause adverse and extremely harmful side effects.

Phenytoin, one of the most prevalent drugs prescribed for this condition, reportedly causes occasional instances of extremely low blood pressure. Therapeutic doses sometimes cause vision problems, while occasionally causing gum problems and endangering fetuses. Also, besides sometimes resulting in lupus, according to some reports, Phenytoin has also been blamed for a wide variety of skin problems and a possible increase in suicidal thoughts--while decreasing bone density.

Other drugs commonly prescribed for epilepsy, including Carbamazepine and Valproate, also generate a chance for unique and extremely negative side effects.

Amazingly all of these drugs had been thoroughly studied and eventually approved by the U.S. Food and Drug Administration, which has close ties to the multi-billion dollar pharmaceutical industry. These dangerous, expensive and often-ineffective unnatural drugs were approved for use by patients who receive legal prescriptions from physicians.

Although aware of these extreme dangers involving "standard, unnatural drugs," the American Epilepsy Society still has the audacity to target cannabis by proclaiming that it "does not support (that the) use of marijuana for treatment of seizures" is effective.

Additional Issues Surfaced

Numerous additional issues surfaced, as if all these many problems were not already enough to bog down efforts to legalize medicinal marijuana nationwide on the federal level. Controversies relate to the sharply increasing demand for the Charlotte's Web cannabis strain. Among challenges:

Transportation: Moving marijuana across state lines is a serious federal crime, so many patients desperately needing the drug felt that their only viable option was to move to jurisdictions that allow this natural remedy.

Single Location: For the first several years after it initially became super-popular, Charlotte's Web was available only in Colorado, the only state where large quantities of the strain were produced. Advocates of the strain eventually were able to offer this coveted variety in a handful of other states including California.

Reliability and Safety: Because the quality and potency of cannabis often varies sharply--even in cases where specific strains are involved--consumers and physicians had reliability and safety concerns.

Self-Medication: Some consumers using medicinal marijuana and their families complained that they needed to use a "trial-and-error" process, in order to determine the ideal doses. This challenge resulted partly from the fact that potency and overall quality varies. In addition, in many cases there is no agreed-upon "universal way" for patients to take marijuana when attempting to address specific types of medical conditions.

Entourage Effect: Cannabis users and producers determined that in many instances when used for medical purposes the drug is ineffective unless it has a quality called the "entourage effect." This entails using plants that contain certain percentages of cannabis sativa and cannabis indica, plus specific amounts of THC. In some instances marijuana products containing only THC failed to effectively treat certain medical conditions, while cannabis containing only cannabinoid (CBD) also failed. Having the "entourage effect," specific mixtures or percentages of these characteristics is necessary for any positive medicinal results.

Federal standards: Further complicating matters, some advocates of medicinal marijuana from the Democrat Party have hinted that they want the federal government to "fully regulate, monitor and manage" the use, production and distribution of the substance nationwide. In the view of some people, such an outcome would emerge as a "virtual horror story," largely because--they say--the inept and corrupt federal government should refrain from telling people how to live. The significant and steadily increasing numbers of severe management issues involving Obamacare have been cited as prime examples.

Potency increases: Thanks primarily to consistent and expert work over several decades to develop vastly increased THC levels in individual marijuana plants, the average cannabis products sold today are vastly more potent than during the 1960s through the 1970s. At the height of the so-called "Hippie Generation" during the Vietnam War, the vast majority of marijuana sold primarily in the underground market contained THC content as low as 1 percent. By comparison, the average marijuana sold today reportedly contains 17 percent to around 21 percent THC, and sometimes as high as 25 percent or even more. Some people opposed to recreational and medicinal cannabis argue that this increase in potency makes marijuana far more dangerous than alcohol, while others sharply disagree.

Offshore growth: Due to the U.S. federal prohibition against marijuana, numerous research firms and medicinal cannabis companies have started growing and testing specific strains in other countries. Meanwhile, these entrepreneurs or their representatives urge U.S. federal officials to review the results of research on those plants and also the findings of any studies on treating patients. All this is done as the growers strive to generate crops "predictably the same," with universally equal attributes such as the levels of THC, and the percentages of sativa and indica within each plant. This way, when and if those cannabis products eventually reach consumers, physicians and patients ideally would be able to "reasonably believe" that they're dealing with a reliable medication that has specific and healthful attributes.

Home-based Gardeners: Increasing numbers of people apparently are growing their own marijuana in order to sharply minimize costs. The price of cannabis can reach $2,000 to $5,000 or even more per pound. The fee usually hinges on the quality, strain, availability and region where the product is sold. This holds true especially in the "underground" illegal market. But prices also can reach steep levels even when purchased in states allowing recreational marijuana, and often when bought through licensed dispensaries for medicinal purposes. To learn how to effectively grow potent cannabis some novices first learn the basic techniques via magazines or Websites provided by services such as "High Times." People who grow their "own weed" need to realize that doing so is at their own risk; remember that growing, possessing and using cannabis remains a felonious class-one felony under federal law.

Beverages: Entrepreneurs began selling marijuana-infused beverages as high-energy drinks in Colorado, beginning shortly after that state legalized the drug for recreational use. By mid-spring of 2015, however, at least one of the firms, Dixie Elixirs & Edibles, had to modify its packaging in order to conform with rules updated by the state, according to online news reports. The firm needed several months to eliminate a screw-top aluminum bottles; those were replaced with resealable, child-proof packaging that enables users to use a plastic cup for pouring a single dose. Analysts concluded that packaging had quickly emerged as a safety issue in states or jurisdictions that had legalized medicinal marijuana. These necessary updates emerged as very expensive for licensed marijuana sales firms, which focused on creating packages similar to what consumers typically see at grocery stores, pharmacies and beauty shops.

False Memories: A story published by the "London Daily Mail" in April 2013 described scientific research indicating that frequent marijuana users may have false memories--perceiving an environment where they "live in their own reality." Among the study's many negative conclusions: people using marijuana have a less active hippocampus, at least as shown by brain scan results; the hippocampus serves as as a person's vital center for storing and retrieving memories; and several months after people in the study group stopped smoking their memory problems continued. Just as disturbing, the study concluded that marijuana can sometimes trigger memories of events that never actually occurred; "mistakes" such as these most often happen among aging people or individuals suffering from psychiatric disorders.

5
Basic Details About Marijuana

Although most famous for causing psychoactive effects commonly known as "the high," marijuana also generates numerous changes within the human body.

Besides the well-known "psychological effects" from getting high, bodily effects impact the "physiological" realm; these impact numerous major organ systems. Among the most common effects or symptoms:

Eyes: The eyes often redden while intra-ocular pressure decreases.

Mouth: The mouth often becomes dry, in some cases extensive.

Sensations: The basic senses of taste, touch, and smell are enhanced. The skin becomes extremely sensitive to cold and heat.

Cardiac: The heart rate increases, although rarely to extremely dangerous levels.

Tension: Muscles relax throughout the body as stress subsides.

Nausea: Any nausea or vomiting that a person suffers immediately before taking marijuana invariably decreases or disappears. The drug also prevents nausea for limited periods.

Pain: Marijuana relieves, controls and manages pain. Most psychoactive cannabis users consider the drug far more powerful than standard analgesics.

Appetite: Much of the time the person's appetite intensifies, sometimes generating an intense hunger typically called "the munchies."

Marijuana Prices

The price of marijuana varies significantly worldwide, according to a wide variety of surveys, law enforcement data and news reports.

Officials generally seem to agree that prices usually hinge on availability coupled with the perceived psychoactive strength of the available "product."

Needless to say, a marijuana crop yielding weak buds that generate an indiscernible high will get low-dollar in the public marketplace; tremendous highs get top-dollar.

Added to this mix is the inescapable fact that an overabundance of cannabis products in a particular community or region often results in price reductions.

Conversely, in instances where cannabis is in extremely limited supply or difficult to find the price generally increases, sometimes to significant levels.

According to a 2008 report by ABC News, at the time authorities deemed marijuana the fourth most valuable crop in the United States. Journalists and pro-cannabis organizations estimated the average nationwide street value at $3,000 per pound.

As of 2008, the United Nations Office on Drugs and Crime estimated that typical U.S. prices hovered from $280 to $420 per ounce.

Needless to say, marijuana has become a multi-billion-dollar annual industry. This is stunning, particularly when considering the fact that the drug remains illegal under federal law.

Potency Increased

Authorities have differing opinions on whether the average marijuana sold today is far more powerful than typical cannabis sold in the 1960s, as many people claim.

The supposed "word on the street" today insists that significant advances in marijuana cultivation during the past five decades have sharply increased potency.

Before the late 1960s, authorities and users of the drug never knew that the "high" primarily comes from flowers of female cannabis plants.

Once that discovery was made, entrepreneurs working in

the underground market developed numerous ways to enhance the buds and remove males plants. These various factors, in turn, supposedly super-charged the average potency in the open marketplace.

Although officials and consumers seem to disagree on these overall factors, an undeniable fact remains. Highly potent marijuana is readily available nationwide.

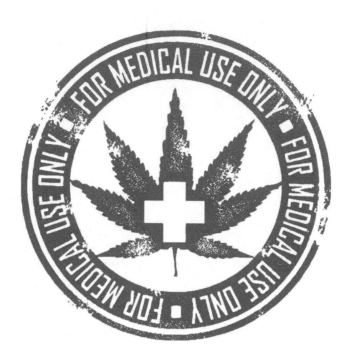

6
Medical Marijuana

The aforementioned fact that many people use "medical marijuana" as a bogus or fraudulent excuse for abusing the drug remains an urgent concern nationwide.

Yet physicians and millions of patients have correctly identified many highly effective and legitimate medical uses for psychoactive cannabis.

The term "medical marijuana" refers to instances where physicians or health experts prescribe the drug as an herbal remedy for specific ailments.

Despite such claims, on a worldwide scale the prescribing of marijuana for medical use has been limited to only a handful of countries.

Besides numerous states within the USA, medical marijuana is legal in Spain, the Netherlands, Canada, Australia and Belgium. Pro-marijuana advocates insist that the number of countries or jurisdictions that allow medical cannabis is likely to grow.

In most jurisdictions that allow medical marijuana, a prescription is required while local laws dictate permissible distribution methods.

Extensive History of Medical Use

Numerous books and media reports claim that the use of marijuana for medical purposes has been underway for several thousand years.

Since long before Christ many cultures have used cannabis for a wide variety of ailments, everything from controlling pain to relieving stress or anxiety.

For the most part until the early 1900s the drug remained widely used for medical purposes on a widespread international scale.

Yet this suddenly slowed during the 20th Century within the United States. Mainstream medical industry professionals feared that any widespread use and legalization of the drug would threaten their professions.

Even today, the primary mainstream medical industry within the USA still opposes any widespread legalization of cannabis for medicinal purposes.

In recent years organizations that have opposed medical marijuana have included the American Medical Association, and the American Society of Addiction Medicine.

Other medical groups have tried to delay the widespread legalization of medical marijuana. For instance, the American Academy of Pediatrics insists that much more study is needed on the issue, although the organization admits cannabinoids may have legitimate uses for medical therapy.

Streams of Studies Results Exist

Contrary to claims by medical organizations that "much more study is needed," extensive scientific research on marijuana has been conducted in recent decades. The bulk of this research has been done outside the United States. In almost every instance these reports indicate that marijuana generates substantial benefits for a wide variety of medical conditions.

Even so, within the USA highly trained medical experts seem to agree that they lack an overall consensus on marijuana's long-term effects on the human body.

Most scientists and doctors would like to see much more detail on the long-term impact generated by psychoactive cannabis on memory and cognitive abilities.

The worry here comes down to the fact that scientists still lack irrefutable data on whether the continual use of marijuana over extended periods injures brain function.

Authorities also want to know much more about the short- and long-term impacts of marijuana on teenagers, and particularly children who accidentally use the drug.

Mainstream Opposition Continues

Pro-marijuana advocates insist that on a broad scale cannabis is extremely safe for adults to use regularly, particularly for medical purposes.

Even so, the U.S. Food and Drug Administration, which as previously stated has close ties to major drug companies, joins mainstream medical organizations in opposing the drug.

This bureaucratic problem has become so pervasive that the FDA has refrained from authorizing naturally grown, wild psychoactive cannabis plants for any type of medical use.

Such intentional oversights strike many practitioners of natural medicine as offensive, while federal officials favor the huge drug industry nicknamed "Big Pharma."

The bureaucrats want to force consumers to avoid natural remedies, while instead requiring them to use harmful, expensive and potentially addictive synthetic drugs.

The "War" Against Consumers Continues

In essence, by blocking marijuana for medicinal use on a nationwide scale, federal authorities have declared an all-out war against consumers who yearn for this effective, generally safe natural remedy--often "affordable" when compared to synthetic drugs.

The "feds" are fighting on behalf of Big Pharma, which essentially are "legally operating" the biggest, most profitable drug ring.

On the other side of battle lines are pro-marijuana organizations and consumers who insist that cannabis works far better, safer and at a lower cost than standard drugs.

The resulting conflict has literally erupted into an all-out "peaceful war," actually a modern-day domestic "cold war" where everyone essentially ends up losing--at least somewhat:

consumers "lose" because they are denied a natural substance that genuinely helps them; covert marijuana harvesters "lose" because they remain on the run or imprisoned due to senseless federal law that makes the possession, use, growing or sale of the drug a felony; and taxpayers lose, forced to fund billions of dollars for the "War on Drugs," which many officials admit is misguided and unwinnable.

Stop the Political Nonsense

Envision a situation where consumers across the USA can readily get medicinal marijuana, while doctors still eagerly prescribe dangerous, expensive drugs.

Within any ideal or "Utopia" situation officials would give both sides on this issue free-reign to do what they want--but that is unlikely to ever happen within the "real world."

You see, within the American political system money and power reign supreme.

Right now those necessary attributes for political clout are held by Big Pharma, and inept politicians who eagerly accept super-high campaign contributions from drug companies.

While the United States arguably has the world's best political system, such corruption remains pervasive on a widespread and seemingly unshakable scale.

Remember that Big Pharma has many billions of dollars to spend controlling such issues, essentially manipulating government and lawmakers to its political whims.

All along, for the most part pro-marijuana groups fail to come anywhere close to amassing such funds necessary for making significant changes on the political front.

Target their Weakness

Determined to move forward with their political battle, the pro-medicinal marijuana crowd has targeted the apparent weaknesses of Big Pharma and its allies.

The key to success here for medical marijuana users lies in local and state politics, where Big Pharma and congressional politicians seem to have less clout.

Using this strategy, the sensible and meticulous pro-marijuana organizations have been able to steadily implement state and regional legalization regulating medicinal marijuana.

Observing this confrontation has emerged into somewhat like watching sports on television. With increased frequency in recent years this evolution has been reported in underground Websites and across the mainstream news media.

Sadly, average consumers seem to lack any inkling that the real behind-the-scenes players here actually are The Politicians and Big Pharma--verses the "so-called little guy."

"Private Money" Plays a Role

Until recently Big Pharma wielded the so-called upper-hand, made possible by continually using a chunk of its automatic ongoing revenue to push authorities into maintaining and expanding the federal War on Drugs.

Since the 21st Century began, opponents of Big Pharma who advocate legalizing medicinal and recreational marijuana have generated big bucks as well--although at far lower levels than their political adversaries.

The pro-marijuana crowd has been increasingly successful, backed by donations from consumers who demand full legal access to the drug.

As the age-old saying goes, "money talks." Hugh income potential is on the line for a steadily increasing number of companies that legally produce and sell marijuana.

Other entrepreneurial ventures that stand to earn big bucks include private "mom-and-pop" medicinal marijuana venues that operate on a local or statewide basis.

Indeed, lots of budding cannabis industry entrepreneurs have much to lose and a lot to gain, the outcome depending largely on who wins on the political battlefront.

Civil War Comparisons

Comparisons between the current legal marijuana battles and the American Civil War of the 1860s become difficult to ignore.

Historians place much of the credit for the North's victory on its greater abundance of vital resources as compared to the outmatched South.

The Union led by Commander-and-Chief and President Abraham Lincoln benefited from its greater manpower, coupled with a mighty industrial war machine.

In a sense today's inept Washington politicians, the FDA and Big Pharma are allied together as the proverbial equivalent of the mighty North. They have far more money and political clout than their adversaries.

All along, somewhat like armies of the rebellious South, modern advocates of medicinal marijuana and legalized cannabis lack the money, infrastructure, manpower and overall clout of their adversaries.

Largely as a result, the current political battle has evolved into "guerrilla warfare," where pro-marijuana advocates intermittently attack on a hit-and-miss basis. Some sporadic victories have resulted, as psychoactive cannabis ventures intermittently become legalized on a state, local or municipal basis.

"Live Free or Die"

Primarily because of their ever-changing guerrilla strategies, pro-marijuana advocates have become the proverbial equivalent of original American revolutionaries.

Today's supporters of marijuana have a "live free or die" attitude, much like those early warriors who supported the American Declaration of Independence.

Unlike early revolutionaries, however, today's political warriors fighting for medicinal marijuana lack any famous leaders who boast household-name status.

On July 4, 1776, the revolution's famous leaders included the likes of George Washington, Thomas Jefferson and John Adams-- all popular in their day.

Yet most of today's consumers who eagerly want recreational or medicinal marijuana apparently would be hard-pressed to name a single person or organization fighting for their cause.

Complex and interlinking political and economic confrontations such as this have generated unpredictable outcomes throughout human history. Thus, predicting the long-term outcome or eventual results of these efforts becomes a coin-toss at best.

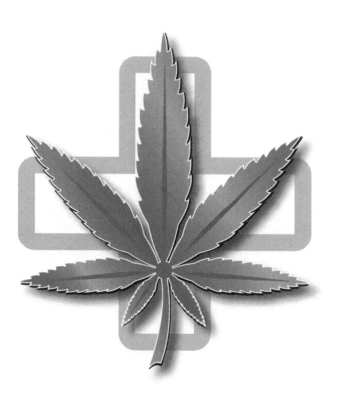

7

Marijuana's Irrefutable Medical Benefits

While the debate on medicinal marijuana continues, authorities need to acknowledge that numerous medical studies--most conducted outside the United States--have confirmed the many positive medical benefits of marijuana.

Such findings sharply contrast the conclusions reached by organizations such as the National Institute on Drug Abuse. Funded by the federal government, just like the FDA, the institute has concluded that marijuana is "an unlikely medication candidate."

Ludicrous and incorrect statements such as these serve as proof that federal bureaucrats consider today's consumers as mere fools, unable to make good choices.

Streams of seemingly endless non-stop declarations by medicinal marijuana users everywhere signal that federal authorities are actually the "most misinformed people."

Consumers have become much more difficult to deceive, thanks to today's instant technology and information-sharing systems that range from text messaging and email to blogs and social networks.

The type of deceptive propaganda that worked on the masses of Russia and China when those nations became communist in the first half of the 20th Century would fail today--at least any efforts to universally convince everyone that "marijuana is totally bad and useless."

For as long as consumers have access to these rapid-fire "free speech" communication systems, a large percentage of them will want, need and demand medicinal marijuana.

Accept and Acknowledge Benefits

Officials need to acknowledge and accept the irrefutable fact that people are becoming increasingly aware of marijuana's many amazing medicinal benefits.

Perhaps best of all, as previously stated, at least from the perspective of many cannabis users the drug never generates long-term negative side effects.

Almost weekly and even daily in recent years scientists have been proclaiming new positive discoveries regarding medicinal cannabis.

Also on the positive side, as they ponder possible recreational and medicinal marijuana laws, state and local lawmakers in growing numbers of jurisdictions have been increasingly willing to consider these scientific findings.

To their credit, this is why growing numbers of states are steadily beginning to adopt laws allowing medicinal marijuana or modifying their regulations in order to expand the number of permissible uses of the drug.

Nausea and Vomiting Issues

As a physician specializing in mainstream and alternative cancer treatment methods, I know first-hand that marijuana-based products significantly alleviate two of the most destructive symptoms induced by standard chemotherapy.

Poisonous chemo made by Big Pharma to kill cancer--as well as healthy cells throughout the body--invariably causes nausea and vomiting. Cannabis effectively eliminates, prevents or controls these unwanted and torturous symptoms.

According to a 2013 article in "Pharmacotherapy," studies prove that cannabis is somewhat effective in treating these symptoms.

Additional scientific studies have declared marijuana is a "reasonable option" for cancer patients whose nausea and vomiting fail to improve with conventional drugs.

60

Even more promising, according to another study released in 2012, cannabis proved more effective than standard pharmaceuticals in treating these adverse symptoms.

On the negative side, however, at least according to various other scientific papers, in some instances cannabis treatments for nausea and vomiting had to be discontinued due to common side effects of marijuana--hallucinations, dysphoria and dizziness. Also on the negative side, according to a 2012 issue of in "Pharmacotherapy," a study concluded that long-term marijuana use sometimes actually causes nausea and vomiting.

Despite such findings, although their mainstream oncologists might recommend otherwise, all cancer patients should be allowed to choose marijuana as a treatment option when and if experiencing nausea during chemotherapy regimens.

All consumers need to remain pro-active, ready to make decisions based on their own unique needs and symptoms.

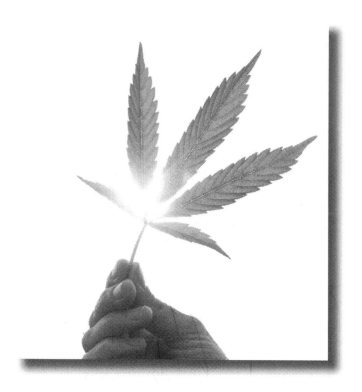

8
Marijuana's Many Medicinal Qualities

Consumers and international scientific researchers have identified countless medicinal health benefits made possible by marijuana.

The list keeps growing at an exponential rate, although mainstream medical professionals almost universally ignore or refuse to acknowledge this important data.

Among some of the related issues and the most promising specific ailments or medical conditions that marijuana "cures" or effectively treats:

HIV and AIDS

Scientists seem to have sharply conflicting opinions on whether marijuana effectively treats adverse symptoms of HIV and AIDS.

Many researchers believe cannabis helps to relive the pain suffered by such patients, while significantly increasing appetites as their body weight drops.

Another focus of attention here concerns whether the psychoactive effects or "high" from marijuana can alleviate or ease mental anguish suffered by such patients.

Whatever the case, getting stoned can at least mildly provide "far more help than damage," particularly among patients in advanced stages of the illness.

Amid these controversial studies, some researchers insist any negative findings should be considered as "suspect" or "unreliable." All AIDS patients have vastly different symptoms and various levels in the advancement of the disease.

These variables become difficult to quantify or accurately

monitor during any attempt at accurate scientific studies, some with insufficient long-term data, inadequate sample sizes, and biases in how the research is performed.

Pain Management

Numerous studies including research reported in 2011 by the "British Journal of Clinical Pharmacology," indicate that cannabis is highly effective in treating chronic non-cancerous pain.

As previously mentioned, for thousands of years people in diverse cultures worldwide have used marijuana to quickly, safely and effectively alleviate pain.

This is critically important, largely because the vast majority of pain medications sold by Big Pharma are highly destructive to the body, sometimes resulting in addiction.

Perhaps best of all from the standpoint of many medicinal marijuana users, the drug often effectively treats debilitating pain caused by nerve-destroying neuropathy.

Many users of medicinal cannabis also insist that marijuana hails as the only substance providing relief from pain caused by rheumatoid arthritis and fibromyalgia.

Yet once again scientific disputes have emerged on the marijuana-pain issue. A 2009 report in "Pain Medicine" indicated that researchers lack any conclusions on whether the apparent benefits of taking cannabis for pain are greater than the risks.

Generating completely opposite findings, a 2011 report in the "British Journal of Clinical Pharmacology" described a study indicating that marijuana is generally safe for use in treating pain. Additionally, according to a 2011 article in "The American Journal of Hospice and Palliative Care," marijuana seems safer in treating pain than opiate-based drugs such as morphine and heroin.

Treating Neurological Issues

At least according to a 2014 article published in "Neurology," doctors and regulatory officials still lack definitive conclusions on whether marijuana effectively treats neurological disorders like epilepsy, multiple sclerosis, and movement problems.

Researchers also say their various studies have been inconclusive on whether cannabis effectively treats the numerous adverse symptoms of multiple sclerosis.

Even so, a 2009 article in "BMC Neurology" said that extracts of cannabidiol and the THC psychoactive ingredient of marijuana provided relief from spasticity--a negative symptom of diseases like "spastic cerebral palsy," a common form of cerebral palsy.

If these findings are correct, however, using marijuana for short periods might fail to provide long-term relief from spasticity that causes an unusual pull, tightness or stiffness of muscles.

The study reported by "BMC Neurology" said that researchers failed to find significant, permanent changes in spasticity of such patients who used marijuana.

Later, generating paradoxical and conflicting results often typical throughout the science, another report described in an April 2014 issue of "Neurology" described a study where cannabis extract taken orally reduced the spasticity suffered by such patients.

Almost as if adding additional intrigue to these overall challenges, a 2013 report in "Pharmacotherapy" indicated that a "trial use" of cannabis would be a reasonable option for patients who first tried mainstream drugs that ultimately failed.

Cannabis-Based Drugs

Although overall the FDA seems somewhat biased against marijuana, at least the agency has approved cannabis for use in two different brand-name drugs. They are:

Dronabinol: Listed as a Schedule III drug illegal to use, distribute, or sell in non-prescription form under federal law, this is sold under the brand name Marinol. Doctors can prescribe this as an "antiemetic" used primarily to treat nausea and vomiting induced by chemotherapy. This drug also can be used to stimulate appetite.

Nabilone: Sometimes sold under the brand name Cesamet, physicians also can prescribe this to treat nausea and vomiting caused by chemo.

Mainstream doctors prescribe Marinol or Cesamet only after conventional treatments fail to address the vomiting and nausea caused by chemotherapy.

Scientists also have developed another cannabis-based prescription drug, but those pills were only available in 2013 outside the United States in Canada, Australia and eight European countries.

Nabiximols is sold under the brand name Sativex, used to control intractable cancer pain and also for minimizing or controlling the adverse conditions of neuropathic pain and spasticity caused by multiple sclerosis.

As of a 2013 article published in "Pharmacotherapy," clinical trials for the possible U.S. approval of Sativex were underway-- under observation by the FDA.

Additional reports have indicated that the effectiveness of these drugs is somewhat challenging to monitor because they are taken orally. Cannabis administered this way takes longer to enter the blood system, in some cases several hours--a sharp contrast to the instant application when inhaling the drug.

Cannabis Treatment for Cancer

According to a 2013 story in "Health Canada," laboratory experiments indicated that psychoactive cannabis has anti-tumor and anti-carcinogenic attributes. These positive characteristics also might assist in the fight against breast and lung cancers.

Other articles published in 2012 revealed that scientists have conducted little formal research on marijuana's possible effectiveness in treating people with the disease.

A disturbing development occurred in November 2013 when

the National Cancer Institute admitted in its own reports that the organization was unaware of any clinical trials on the potential effectiveness of marijuana byproducts in treating cancer. The Institute mentioned only one small study indicating that the psychoactive THC might fight or prevent cancerous tumors.

A 2013 article in "Cancer Research UK" contended that scientists lack firm evidence that using marijuana prevents cancer. Researchers insist that such data is difficult to quantify and reach conclusions from, primarily because a large percentage of cannabis users also smoke tobacco--an extremely dangerous carcinogen.

(Despite these conflicting claims, please see Chapter X on how "cannabis oil" has been used to "cure," eliminate or control cancer.)

Dementia and Alzheimer's Disease

Some researchers believe that marijuana can play a significant role in managing or slowing the development of Alzheimer's Disease, according to numerous stories in early 2015 throughout the mainstream news media.

Even so, other reports as recently as 2012 by the Royal Society of London concluded that a review on the possible effectiveness of cannabinoids in treating the aging of the brain is "either inconclusive or still missing."

Adding disappointment to those eager for an Alzheimer's cure, in 2009 a report by the independent, non-government, non-profit Cochran Collaboration reached negative conclusions. The report stated that only one controlled, randomized trial had been conducted in an effort to determine the effectiveness of marijuana in treating dementia.

The organization said that the results were poorly presented, while failing to provide "sufficient data to draw any useful conclusions."

Even so, in September 2014 the "Journal of Alzheimer's

Disease" published a research report strongly suggesting that THC could be a "potential therapeutic treatment option for Alzheimer's Disease through multiple functions and pathways."

Additional positive news came in March 2015 when LSU Health New Orleans agreed to support the Utah-based CB Biosciences startup company's research into developing cannabis-based products for effectively treating Alzheimer's and Parkinson's.

The report said that the company agreed to make an initial $428,000 investment to support ongoing research by Doctor Chu Chen. Under the agreement the company will license any products that the doctor develops.

Potential Diabetes Treatments

According to the "Handbook of Experimental Pharmacology," cannabidiol from marijuana might slow the damaging of vital bodily cells sometimes caused by diabetes mullites type 1.

Even so, as noted by the "British Journal of Diabetes and Vascular Disease," researchers have been unable to find any meaningful evidence regarding marijuana's possible effectiveness on people suffering from diabetes.

A 2010 review by the Society concluded that "the potential risks and benefits for diabetic patients remain unquantified at the present time."

Contrary to this report, however, a 2015 article by "The Daily Chronic" described a French study that has linked marijuana use to a lower risk of diabetes in HIV/AIDS patients.

In addition, the story said, "a history of cannabis use is positively associated with a lower risk of insulin resistance" in such patients.

Meantime, although doctors lack in-depth research on marijuana's possible effectiveness in treating diabetes, many people with the disease insist that cannabis controls and minimizes their pain.

Marijuana for Glaucoma

Many people suffering from glaucoma, a dreaded disease causing blindness unless successfully treated, claim that medicinal marijuana provides them with significant help.

For several decades doctors and researchers have known with certainty that marijuana relieves intraocular pressure in the eye. This becomes a critically important factor because excessive eye pressure is the primary negative symptom of glaucoma.

Even so, the American Glaucoma Society discourages marijuana use by people with the disease. The organization cites two reasons.

First, any relief in intraocular pressure is only short-term, ending when the effects of the drug wear off.

And secondly, according to the society, researchers have been unable to confirm whether marijuana alters the course of the disease.

Despite such claims, I know a glaucoma patient who insists that medicinal marijuana has given her significant help in fighting the disease.

"The only times that I can see with my left eye are when I use marijuana," she said. "My mainstream eye doctor refuses to discuss this with me, despite my instance that this is a 'wonder-drug' that he should consider or at least talk about."

Other glaucoma patients agree, including actor and media personality Whoopi Goldberg, who has told reporters she uses marijuana as a glaucoma treatment.

Tourette Syndrome

According to various medical reports, marijuana has potential for addressing the symptoms of Tourette syndrome, an inherited neuropsychiatric condition that generates bothersome physical and vocal tics. Once considered rare and bizarre, this condition sometimes forces sufferers to involuntarily shout obscene words.

A 2009 report in "Lancet Neurology" described a review where Tourette patients lacked serious adverse effects, while also having a beneficial response to Marinol pills containing the psychoactive ingredients of marijuana.

Par for the course, however, according to a 2000 edition of the "Journal of Neurology" a review of separate studies indicated that cannabis increased the inner tension of Tourette sufferers--while failing to eliminate tics.

Completely different findings detailed in a 2009 Cochran review described two control trials involving concentrated THC; that substance had a positive impact on these symptoms. On the negative side, however, the report said that the improvements in tic frequency and severity were small, only detected by "some of the outcome measures."

Sensible Policy Against Prosecution

Whether correct or incorrect some political junkies through the first phase of President Obama's second term had criticized then-Attorney General Eric Holder.

Yet advocates of medicinal cannabis universally applauded one of Holder's most controversial statements, announcing a policy that the U.S. government would refrain from criminally prosecuting anyone who uses medicinal marijuana for legitimate reasons.

Holder proclaimed that "it will not be a priority to use federal resources to prosecute patients with serious illnesses, or their caregivers who are complying with state laws on medicinal marijuana."

On the opposite side of the political spectrum, though, Holder also promised that "we will not tolerate drug traffickers who hide behind claims of compliance with state law to mask activities that are clearly illegal."

Such statements seem to have lessened at least some concerns of medicinal marijuana users. They had feared that federal officials would behave like tough old American west lawmen, trampling on the supposed rights of ill people nationwide who want to use and benefit from medicinal marijuana.

The Legal Fight Continues

People who want medicinal marijuana legalized nationwide are waging a separate political battle from those striving to approve the drug's recreational use nationwide.

Two separate non-profit companies are helping to lead the way in pushing for the nationwide legalization of medical cannabis. Medical Marijuana Inc., and Cannabis Science Inc., share the mutual goal of helping more patients benefit from the drug.

A primary goal of each of these companies focuses on convincing the FDA to approve cannabis-based medicines, including inhaled marijuana.

This way, as hoped by Cannabis Science Inc., everyone nationwide will have access to medicinal marijuana wherever they live.

Simultaneously, a third organization, The Multidisciplinary Association for Psychedelic Studies (MAPS), wants FDA approval of medical cannabis for the treatment of post-traumatic stress disorder.

Until the FDA and the federal government loosen marijuana restrictions, U.S. citizens suffering from ailments, who want to benefit from medicinal cannabis, and who live in states without dispensaries of the drug have only two options:

Move: Relocate to states that allow medicinal or recreational cannabis.

Illegal purchases: Buy the drug illegally on the so-called underground or criminal-backed market. We do not recommend this!

The Political Battle Continues Unabated

Streams of pro-marijuana advocates nationwide have

aggressively joined the efforts to legalize medical cannabis. Some of these individuals are relatively famous actors and musicians.

Amazingly, a limited number of congressional representatives and U.S. senators from both mainstream political parties have stood tall in joining individuals and organizations eager for the nationwide legalization of cannabis for recreational and medicinal purposes. The most noteworthy former politicians here have ranged from congressmen Barney Frank, a Democrat, to Ron Paul, a Republican.

Adding a scientific foundation to their efforts, pro-marijuana organizations have been joined by numerous legendary scientists and researchers including Milton Friedman and the late Carl Sagan.

Just as essential, streams of widely acclaimed writers have supported the legalization of medical cannabis. Besides myself, the many authors who support the legalization of medical marijuana have included the late internationally acclaimed author Robert Anton Wilson, and Ann Druyan, co-writer of the popular 1990 PBS documentary "The Cosmos," and its 2014 follow-up, "Cosmos: A Spacetime Odyssey." Druyan is Sagan's widow.

Individually and collectively, many of these authors are actively joining or forming non-profit organizations dedicated to pushing for the legalization of medical cannabis. At present, though, authorities apparently lack any formal estimate on how much money these organizations have collectively spent--or plan to spend--in the ongoing efforts to reach their political goals.

The Anti-Marijuana Crowd

Streams of big-name celebrities, politicians and bureaucrats have eagerly joined organizations that aggressively oppose medicinal marijuana.

Besides controversial conservative nationwide talk-radio host Rush Limbaugh, some of the "biggest names" here include former Republican Presidents George H.W. Bush and his son, "Bush the

Second," George W. Bush.

Former governors who failed in their own presidential bids, but who actively oppose efforts to legalize medicinal marijuana, include Republicans Mitt Romney of Massachusetts, Mike Huckabee of Arkansas, along with current New Jersey Gov. Chris Christie.

Whether merely pandering to their masses within their political base, or legitimately opposed to medical marijuana, so-called big-name celebrities such as these often attract tons of media attention whenever they speak about controversial issues.

This attribute, in turn, serves as a proverbial political lightning rod for energizing anti-marijuana organizations such as the International Narcotics Control Board.

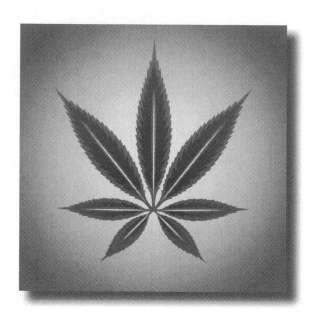

9

Inept Government Inadvertently Admits Cannabis Cures Cancer

In perhaps the most significant news ignored in decades by the liberal mainstream news media, in April 2015 "High Times" magazine issued a story entitled, "Federal Government Unwittingly Admits Cannabis Kills Cancer."

If the nation's primary news outlets ever bothered to reveal these findings, the public's response would be "nothing less than phenomenal"--generating an intense call by people coast-to-coast to fully legalize marijuana for cancer treatment.

This story confirmed by numerous so-called underground online blogs confirmed that the U.S. federal government supports a study concluding that marijuana used to control cancer can destroy the disease.

In April 2015, the U.S. National Institute on Drug Abuse revealed that it supports the findings of the research, conducted by scientists at Saint George's University in London, England. Results of the London study had been announced in November 2014.

What is significantly "new" in this instance is the fact that the U.S. government actually acknowledged and supported the specific positive findings of such a marijuana study.

Numerous other news reports, all that received little mainstream news media attention through the past several decades, have chronicled similar results from other studies about the cannabis. Each concluded that the drug cures cancer.

However, although this development might seem fantastic to advocates supporting medicinal marijuana, a "sad fact remains"-- namely that the government likely will never allow cannabis as a preferred, safe and affordable cancer medicine.

Pot Taxes: The annual federal U.S. income tax filing deadline of April 15 has become a national day of mourning for licensed, legitimate marijuana distribution and sales businesses nationwide. Because the drug is illegal under federal law, these operations are unable to use standard deductions for business expenses, everything from accounting fees to employee wages and much more. In April 2015, the McClatchy News Service reported that these ventures want to change the federal law, which they consider outdated and discriminatory. McClatchy quoted Nick Cihlar, a co-owner of Subdued Excitement Inc., in Washington state, as saying, "We don't want special favors. We just want to be treated like businesspeople." Subdued Excitement sells marijuana products to licensed state retailers. Anti-marijuana advocates claim that allowing tax breaks for marijuana businesses would be a mistake. Some opponents of psychoactive cannabis say that giving such businesses tax breaks would be "audacious" for domestic marijuana companies, which are violating federal law.

Judge Makes Ruling: In a landmark ruling that failed to generate widespread national news coverage, in April 2015 a U.S. federal judge refused to remove marijuana from the country's Schedule I list of the most dangerous drugs. According to the "Los Angeles Times," U.S. District Judge Kimberly J. Mueller declined to remove psychoactive cannabis from the prohibited list of the most dangerous narcotics, which include extremely dangerous and often deadly drugs like LSD and heroin. Mueller declared that she "could not lightly overturn a law passed by Congress," the Times said. The judge's ruling came one year after she agreed to hold an extended hearing on the issue. Appointed by President Obama, Mueller ruled on the constitutionality of listing marijuana on the worst-drugs list; her decision came in response to a pre-trial motion filed by lawyers who represented accused marijuana growers. Lawyers for the defendants said that Mueller's decision could not be appealed until after their trial, expected in early 2016.

Christie Decision: Showing his political ignorance and an ill-advised refusal to carefully study the facts, in April 2015 New Jersey Governor Chris Christie, a Republican, vowed that if elected president "I will crack down and not permit" legalized marijuana. According to various news reports, Christie proclaimed on the "Hugh Hewitt Show" that as president he would "crack down" on states that have legalized marijuana. By issuing this policy, Christie essentially turned his back on medical experts like Doctor Sanjay Gupta. For as long as Americans continue electing politicians with such irresponsible policies, the government will maintain and enforce draconian and out-of-date anti-marijuana laws.

Synthetic Marijuana: At least until such time as marijuana is legalized nationwide, licensed or clandestine companies likely will continue producing and selling extremely dangerous "synthetic pot." In some instances such drugs had been legally sold on a temporary basis in some states, before becoming criminalized in those jurisdictions after officials began realizing the dangers. During the spring of 2015, for instance, according to news reports a drug that mimics marijuana forced 227 people to visit emergency rooms in Mississippi over a two-week period. The previous month, 300 people went to Alabama emergency rooms when suffering from similar symptoms after taking synthetic marijuana. Streams of similar incidents with varying degrees of severity had occurred during the previous decade in many states. Ultimately, some people will strive to get high, even if overly harsh laws remain. And even if marijuana were legalized, entrepreneurs with nefarious intentions likely would continue making dangerous substances that mimic the drug. The cost of buying such products usually is much lower than the street value of psychoactive cannabis.

Support for marijuana surges: The percentage of Americans who want marijuana legalized had sharply increased among key demographic groups by the spring of 2015, according to survey results released by the Pew Research Center. Nationwide support for legalizing cannabis held steady, with 53 percent of people surveyed declaring that they would support such a change. The biggest support by far comes from young adults ages 18 to 34, with an astounding 68 percent of them supporting legalization. The overall support for marijuana comes from people of all ages from both mainstream political parties. The only significant opposition came from conservative Republicans, who oppose marijuana legalization by a 2-to-1 margin. These trends mark a substantial change from the late 1960s and early 1970s, when less than 20 percent of Americans of all ages and political parties told public opinion surveys that they would support marijuana legalization. Overall support for the drug increased as improved communication systems gave consumers better access to important information about marijuana.

Doctors verses Patients

Do instances such as the epilepsy issue signify that mainstream doctors have essentially gone to war against patients? In doing so, are mainstream physicians essentially declaring that "we know what is best for you, mainly because we happen to be doctors, and also because there are no adequate studies on marijuana?"

And are doctors and medical institutions allied with Big Pharma and the FDA taking advantage of the fact that comprehensive, broad-scale studies on the possible medical benefits of marijuana are unlikely to occur--at least in the short term?

Whatever the "best, true" answers might be here becomes irrelevant to patients who insist that they desperately need medical marijuana for their ailments.

With this in mind, what aggressive and sensible moves have the mainstream medical organizations done to push for major unbiased studies regarding marijuana?

At least judging by the lack of news reports about any such

potential efforts, the mainstream medical industry seems to be ignoring the controversy.

Charlotte's Web Issues

Further complicating matters, according to a 2014 "National Journal" article, the precise status remains unclear on whether Charlotte's Web is legal nationwide on a federal basis.

Although at least 23 states allowed at least some form of medical marijuana, this strain had not yet been specifically authorized for medical use in some of those states.

In addition, some state legislatures were considering such authorization, while somewhat similar proposals were being written for future consideration in other jurisdictions.

In a program that Reuters and the CBS Denver affiliate labeled as "pot for tots," New Jersey Governor Chris Christie considered allowing sick children to have access to medical cannabis.

Energized by Colorado's landmark medical cannabis legislation, in July 2014, Republican Congressman Scott Perry of Pennsylvania introduced a bill nicknamed the "Charlotte's Web Medical Hemp Act of 2014." If passed, he said, the new law would amend the Controlled Substances Act, "the federal law that criminalizes marijuana, to exempt plants with an extremely low percentage of THC, the chemical that makes users high."

More Courageous Politicians Needed

Our country needs many more congressmen and senators, and even a president, with enough political courage like that of Representative Perry. Rather than grandstanding or "sitting on the proverbial fence" regarding this issue, our nation's lawmakers need to collectively take a common-sense approach in legalizing marijuana, especially for medical purposes.

All federal agencies that regulate public health issues, along with Congress, also need to take an aggressive leadership role in launching comprehensive, non-biased research into the drug's effectiveness for treating specific ailments.

For this to happen, several actions must occur. Among them:

Leadership: The nation needs a strong leader to make this happen, particularly a president who refrains from taking nebulous and unspecific stances on the issue.

Voters: Citizens must aggressively lobby for passage of such legislation as steadily increasing percentages of the American public demand medical marijuana.

Support: Besides supporting specific candidates who advocate medicinal cannabis, concerned citizens should consider donating to pro-marijuana organizations. (Lots of those groups and their contact information are listed near the back of this book, in Chapter X, immediately before the "Bonus Section" on cancer treatment at Century Wellness Clinic.)

Battle: Remain aware that an arduous, unending "political fight" likely will remain necessary, particularly when opposing medical organizations and candidates that want anti-marijuana laws.

Research: Support political candidates who vow to push for a federal program that gives scientists access to marijuana for research, and also start to approve psychoactive cannabis farms for those scientists.

A collective and consistent effort is needed for the nationwide legalization of medicinal cannabis. Yet this formidable task will be well worth the process, essential for saving lives in some instances, and possibly for improving the overall quality of life for many patients.

Insurance Issues

Users of medicinal marijuana in the United States also face potentially significant financial issues, because insurance companies refuse to pay for drugs that have not been officially approved by the FDA for distribution in prescription form.

The vast majority of health issues effectively addressed by

marijuana target far more ailments and health problems than merely chemo-induced nausea and vomiting.

As a result, once again the federal government has failed consumers, particularly people who insist that marijuana serves as the only effective remedy for their ailments.

Much of the issue comes down to the fact that Obamacare has side-stepped this issue, rather than "doing the right thing" by paying for cannabis needed by patients.

So, does this signal yet another instance where greedy Big Pharma and its incompetent allies in Congress have intentionally overlooked the urgent needs of U.S. citizens?

Even before officials could approve such payments, under federal law the FDA would first need to permit studies on the effectiveness of marijuana--specifically identifying the positives and the negatives.

Some observers correctly surmise that this scenario likely would never happen, because any tests would be merely subjective with a biased favoring Big Pharma.

Medical Marijuana Shops

The number of licensed medical marijuana dispensaries and jurisdictions that legally allow growing cannabis for this purpose changes constantly as various state and regional laws continually evolve.

In 2013, medical marijuana dispensaries and legal, licensed growing were allowed in 23 states and the District of Columbia, according to news reports. Those totals are likely to increase or at least change as more jurisdictions consider such laws.

Amazingly, according to a 2014 article in the "National Post," officials considered allowing "marijuana vending machines"-- possibly in the United States and Canada. These devices, some already in operation, are only available inside secure rooms at licensed pot dispensaries.

As an added security measure, some dispensaries allow all

of their employees to operate the machines after obtaining a fingerprint scan from the patient.

Although the number of jurisdictions allowing medicinal marijuana dispensaries continues to grow, critics complain that some supposed "patients" are merely trying to "game the system" in order to use marijuana for non-medical purposes. Even so, a 2011 article in the "Journal of Psychoactive Drugs" reported that such complaints are difficult to measure.

At virtually all legitimate medicinal marijuana dispensaries, people obtaining the drug must submit a prescription from a licensed doctor or a certified medical professional.

Many of these facilities provide names and addresses of such professionals, and some dispensaries even have licensed medical experts or doctors on their staffs.

International Rules and Product Patents

On an international basis, the number and frequency of licensed medicinal marijuana dispensaries varies significantly-- while still illegal in many nations.

In recent years such stores have been legalized in Spain, the Netherlands, Israel, Finland, Canada, Belgium, Austria, and the United Kingdom. Numerous other nations seem likely to adopt similar rules.

Yet on a worldwide scale such efforts likely would face potential political roadblocks similar to those within the USA.

According to data from the International Narcotics Control Board, cannabis remains categorized as an illegal Schedule IV drug by the United Nations. These antiquated and outdated rules were first adopted in 1961 in Paris at the Single Convention on Narcotic Drugs, an international treaty still in force today.

Officials at the gathering also agreed to resume previously approved harsh classifications for notorious and extremely dangerous drugs like heroin, morphine and cocaine.

Scientists at the time knew relatively little about marijuana, especially the biological attributes of psychoactive cannabis that generate a "high." Since then, largely thanks to the initial findings of scientists in Israel the 1960s, many of today's researchers have concluded that marijuana is much safer than originally believed.

Anti-drug laws and restrictions have historically been imposed in efforts to protect the welfare and health of the general public. A paradoxical situation has emerged, as some people claim that medicinal marijuana helps protect the health and welfare of societies as a whole.

Important Research Remains Stalled

Advancements in marijuana research continue in numerous countries other than the USA. On a gradual basis in recent years some highly respected medical organizations and a handful of groups currently opposed to marijuana have called for further study on the drug.

According to many news reports, these organizations are willing to endorse a reclassification of marijuana in order to conduct further study. They include the American Academy of Family Physicians, the Leukemia and Lymphoma Society, the American College of Physicians, and the American Medical Association.

Statements such as these seem essential in accelerating reliable studies into the effectiveness of medicinal marijuana.

For now, however, American scientists insist that their hands are "essentially tied" because cannabis remains a top-level Schedule I felony under federal law.

As a result, fear of potential prosecution prevents formal, wide-scale and necessary domestic studies regarding the apparent effectiveness of marijuana in treating specific diseases.

Needless to say, this has frustrated many people including some scientists who believe that psychoactive cannabis would be particularly useful in treating severe or fatal ailments such as

Huntington's Disease and Parkinson's Disease.

Bureaucracy Stalls or Blocks Vital Treatment

The various bureaucratic "road bumps and roadblocks" have denied countless people from receiving urgent medicinal marijuana treatments that might help them.

Once again as a society we have essentially allowed government to fail the ailing people among us; they endure needless suffering.

The many diseases and ailments that some scientists insist are effectively treated by marijuana continues to expand as research spreads to other countries.

Exacerbating this tragedy, numerous states that allow medicinal marijuana dispensaries have failed to adopt rules allowing for cannabis treatment for some of these ailments.

10
The Miracle:
How THC Kills Cancer

One of the most famous fantasy dreams for many parents is to have their child "grow up to become the first person to discover a cure for cancer."

Yet amazingly, the most effective natural cure likely has existed for thousands of years, thanks to the THC from marijuana that makes people "high."

As bizarre as this might seem, it's truc--although the vast majority of mainstream doctors and politicians refuse to acknowledge this fact.

Intrigued "weed oil" or "marijuana oil" packed with THC, a handful of scientists and doctors have delved into the question of how this substance kills cancer.

After reviewing the data, as one of the world's most respected oncologists, I have verified how this curative process occurs on a biological and atomic level. The conclusions are both intriguing, mysterious and even undeniably "miraculous."

All along, as a doctor, although such reports are highly encouraging, I refrain from recommending "cannabis oil' for treating cancer until much more thorough study.

Why No Celebration?
If such claims are true, on a basic biological level, this simple, logical and effective method of killing cancer should be a cause for international celebration.

If these sensational details ever got revealed on an instant widespread basis, people would be holding ticker-tape parades worldwide.

Journalists in TV, radio, print and Web media reporting this news would gain as much attention as the end of World War II or when men first landed on the moon.

In an ideal world, backed by our government, mainstream doctors would rush to approve and implement THC as treatment for cancer.

Yet of course, none of this is happening because we live in a corrupt or misguided governmental system where mainstream doctors and hospitals *do not want cancer cured*.

Backed by inept politicians and corrupt bureaucrats, the mainstream medical industry has put up major barriers to keep this vital truth from you.

Imagine the significant drop in their once-gigantic incomes if one of the most dreaded diseases in the history of mankind is suddenly obliterated.

Significant Success Possible

It should go without saying that no medicine should ever be touted as the "greatest snake oil ever created," a guaranteed 100-percent cure for cancer or any other disease.

Even the "Salk" vaccine famously developed in the 1950s to prevent polio has failed to fully eradicate that disease worldwide. Some people, societies and cultures have never had complete access to that highly effective prevention method.

With these essential factors clearly understood, however, the world's medical community and governments need to carefully study and perhaps eventually acknowledge the formidable ability of THC and other basic ingredients from marijuana to obliterate cancer.

"I don't really care about you or your health," mainstream doctors are essentially telling the public, when denying THC's cancer-destroying ability. "I care most about my own pocketbook and my own wealth than your survival."

Without exaggeration, this denial on the part of common, everyday allopathic physicians hails as perhaps by far one of the

86

greatest tragedies in all of human history.

Certainly, today's mainstream medical community is not shoving people into gas chambers by the millions, the way that Nazis did in Europe during World War II.

Sadly, however, the cost of denying this "cure" is just as destructive--or perhaps even more catastrophic than the Holocaust--at least on a broad international human scale.

Many thousands of people perish from cancer worldwide every day, and millions succumb to the disease every year.

By denying the public access to the supposed natural benefits made possible by marijuana oil, the mainstream international medical community is essentially sending many millions of people to their deaths--but only if the "cure" claims are true.

Doctors Behaving Like Robots

Behaving almost as if robots without brains or who lack critical thinking abilities, mainstream doctors keep telling the public that "more study is needed."

Such cowardly behavior hails as the modern equivalent of the Wizard of Oz, who tells his frightened subjects to "pay no attention to the man behind the curtain."

Shockingly but true, the mainstream medical community has repeatedly told the public since the mid-20th Century that much more study is needed on marijuana.

Perhaps worst of all in this regard, the vast majority of people have never heard about the supposedly stupendous curative effects of marijuana oil in effectively treating cancer.

Cleverly, in order to weasel away from the problem, today's allopathic physicians hide behind the fact that the federal government makes marijuana possession a crime.

Because of this restriction, the doctors say, "Our hands are tied; we could not learn the conclusive truth about marijuana--even if we wanted."

This tragedy becomes even more perplexing and downright sad

when acknowledging the fact that the physicians have played a key role in imposing prohibitions against marijuana.

Ceramide Makes the Cure Possible

A little-known waxy lipid that occurs naturally within the human body is called "ceramide." This is the substance that kills the cancer in the following way:

Thriving cancer cells: When healthy and growing fast enough to eventually kill a person, the cells of cancers have only extremely low levels of ceramide. The strong cells of cancer remain vital when those biological structures have minuscule ceramide levels.

THC targets cancer cells: As the psychoactive ingredient of marijuana, THC refrains from attacking the body's normal healthy cells. Instead, the unique characteristics of THC specifically target cancer cells, even those that are initially thriving and healthy.

Cancer cell destruction: Tricky, deceptive and intent on killing the cancer, the THC attaches to the natural CB1 and CB2 receptors on cells of the disease. These are the vital doorways through which THC eventually kills the cancer.

Unique weaponry works: Interacting with the cancer cells' nucleus, the THC forces tiny shifts within the hundreds of thousands of mitochondria. This is a critical phase because mitochondria are necessary for providing cell energy and cell life.

Persistent attacks: When a cancer patient eats marijuana oil multiple times daily, the high THC concentrations effectively interacts with mitochondria and with various organelles within the cancer cell's cytoplasm. Contained within the cell's membrane, the cytoplasm has various internal substructures.

Ceramide build-up: The persistent infusion of THC into the cancer cell increases the levels of ceramide, which then changes the "rheostat" or energy resistance of natural biological structures called "sphingolipids." This compound plays a critical role in the body's natural cell-recognition processes, plus the vital transmission of informational signals among cells.

Cancer cell attacked: The increasing ceramide levels and the changes in sphingolipids within the cancer eventually cause a fatal disruption within the critical mitochondria inside the cell. The mitochondria suffer this "fatal wound" due to structural or "pore permeability" changes in a small hemeprotein called "cytochrome c;" this is a natural internal cellular structure that scientists identify as loosely associated with the inner membrane of mitochondria.

Cancer cell death: As if an NFL quarterback pounded out of the end-zone by a pack of muscular defenders, the natural cytochrome c cellular structure effectively shoves mitochondria from the cancer cell-resulting in the cell's death.

CBD Also Plays Major and Necessary Role

Besides the essential ceramide, the cannabidiol (CBD) elements from marijuana also play an important role in this cancer-curing process.

Additionally, ceramide causes the nucleus of cancer cells to undergo a process that scientists call "genotoxicity;" this condition destroys the chemical agents of cancer cells.

Called "genotoxic stress," the process generates a substance known by a variety of names including "tumor protein p53," "cellular tumor antigen 53," merely "p53" and several other terms. As a vital isoform of a protein, throughout nature "p53" plays a crucial role as a "tumor suppressor" that prevents cancer in multicellular organisms.

Ignited by ceramide increases caused by THC, the additional generation of "p53" disrupts the calcium metabolism of mitochondria within cancer cells.

Adding to THC's firepower in attacking cancer, the ceramide destroys the ability of each cancer cell to digest and benefit from nutrients. To generate this massive attack on each cancer cell's ability to digest nutrients, the ceramide disrupts the cellular "lysosome," a term designating the membrane-bound cell organelle found within most animals.

Cancer Cell Death Becomes a Certainty

Along with various sphingolipids, the ceramide generated by THC actively works to block, inhibit or destroy every biological pathway that cancer needs.

As a result, the ceramide obliterates any chance that the cancer might have to survive. For this to happen, over a period of time the patient needs to consistently take therapeutic amounts of THC and CBD.

To sharply increase the probability for success, this process must start before the "final-days" stage of the patient's life; ideally, the person's THC-CBD regimens should occur without having first undergone chemotherapy or radiation therapy.

By doing so under ideal conditions, without causing undue discomfort or harm to the patient, these combined and controversial ingredients place the cancer cells under continual metabolic pressure. Such ongoing stress obliterates the disease.

Amazingly, the human body has the unique ability to interchangeably use and to benefit from both the THC and CBD.

Ideal THC Content Levels

There are varying opinions on what should be deemed the ideal THC percentages in cannabis oil for treating cancer. Some observers insist that a 60 percent to 70 percent level is OK, while others believe that the best outcomes by far occur when the oil contains 80 percent THC, with the remaining 20 percent containing CBD.

11

The Numerous
Beneficial Powers of THC

As previously mentioned, marijuana often generates hunger that cannabis users often affectionately or casually call "The Munchies."

Many marijuana users apparently fail to realize that these hungers actually are generated primarily by the THC that creates a psychoactive high.

Among the numerous interworking factors that THC uses to create hunger:

Palatability: While generating marijuana's famous "high," THC also interacts with the body's CB1 receptors to enhance food tastes and the positive sensations of eating.

Hunger Hormone: While enhancing taste sensations, the THC simultaneously accelerates the body's natural hunger hormone that scientists call "Ghrelin."

Brain Messages: When the stomach is empty, Ghrelin naturally sends a message to the brain: "I'm hungry." THC sometimes makes this happen even when food is already present within the stomach.

Blocked Messages: After eating a full meal, the body's "Leptin" hormone normally tells the brain: "I'm full." But THC blocks this signal.

Pleasure Factor: Some scientists also believe THC enhances the "hedonistic pleasure" of eating, according to a 2011 article in "Neuropharmacology."

THC Addresses Neurological Disorders
Marijuana and specifically the THC from cannabis addresses

numerous neurological issues, according to a 2014 report by the American Academy of Neurology.

Upon issuing its report, the Academy said its review centered on the safety and effectiveness of marijuana-derived products and of medical marijuana.

The Academy's findings were based on 34 separate studies, generating evidence that THC and cannabis extracts effectively treat serious multiple sclerosis symptoms--and also health issues generated by numerous other neurological diseases.

These findings should be considered significant, partly because the Academy founded in 1948 represents 21,000 currently practicing neurologists and neuroscientists.

With headquarters in Minneapolis, Minnesota, the Academy strives to improve the science and methods for treating serious neurological problems.

Address Multiple Sclerosis Symptoms

The Academy determined that marijuana and THC effectively treat devastating symptoms of multiple sclerosis--sometimes called "MS," a dreaded disease that damages cells in the brain and spinal cord.

The many negative signs and symptoms of MS include physical, mental and even psychiatric problems. Some symptoms relapse or increase over time.

As identified by the Academy, some severe MS symptoms that marijuana and THC effectively treat are:

Painful spasms: Sometimes accompanied by "centrally mediated pain," oral cannabis extract was deemed effective in four low-quality--and four separate high-quality--trials. Researchers also determined that THC is likely effective in treating this debilitating symptom.

Spasticity: MS sometimes causes skeletal muscle performance to deteriorate, generating sensations of tightness, pulling or severe stiffness. Numerous studies rated oral cannabis as effective, and THC "probably effective" in alleviating these symptoms.

Bladder issues: Studies using oral cannabis and THC indicated that these drugs are likely ineffective in attempts to treat bladder problems caused by MS.

Studies Generate Differing Results

Studies have generated differing results on whether cannabis and THC effectively treat other neurological disorders including Alzheimer's and Huntington's diseases. Among the conflicting results:

Alzheimer's disease: A scientific report published in September 2014 in the "Journal of Alzheimer's Disease" said that research strongly suggests that TCH "could be a potential therapeutic treatment option for Alzheimer's disease through multiple functions and pathways." If true, such conclusions could emerge as significant, partly because Alzheimer's is the sixth leading cause of death in the United States--costing the nation's economy an estimated $203 billion annually. Yet in separate research, a 2011 Cochran Review report failed to find significant evidence that cannabis products effectively treat the disease. Scientists likely will disagree on the possible effectiveness of cannabis in treating Alzheimer's, the discussion lasting for many years until more conclusive research results are amassed.

Huntington's disease: As reported by the Academy, scientists were unable to reach conclusions on the possible effectiveness of THC and oral cannabis extract in the treatment of Huntington's disease. However, some advocates of medicinal marijuana disagree with this conclusion. As reported by the "Medical Jane" publication that supports using marijuana for medical purposes, scientists have failed to find a cure for Huntington's--although medications help manage symptoms. People with this ultimately fatal inherited disease suffer from numerous negative symptoms that include behavioral challenges, mood swings and irritability.

"Medical Jane" reports that cannabinoid therapy "reduces Huntington's-like symptoms in mice."

Other Neurological Ailments: The Academy also reports that its researchers have been unable to find conclusive evidence that THC and oral cannabis extract effectively treat numerous other neurological disorders. These include epilepsy, Tourette syndrome and an extremely painful neck disorder called "Spasmodic Torticollis"--sometimes called "Cervical Dystonia." As reported by the "Cincinnati Business Courier" in March 2015, scientists at the University of Cincinnati and the Cincinnati Children's Hospital Medical Center were still investigating medical marijuana as a potential treatment for epilepsy. Specifically, the "Courier" said, rather than using THC, researchers focused on the Epidiolex drug derived from the non-psychoactive cannabidiol extract of marijuana. Meantime, numerous states through 2015 dropped or rejected proposals to add Tourette syndrome to the list of ailments authorized for treatment by cannabis. However, contrary to reports indicating that marijuana lacks effectiveness in treating Tourette, some people continued insisting that the disease should be listed as a permissible condition for medical marijuana treatment.

12
Meet the "Heroes"

Cannabis expert Constance Finley of Northern California has rapidly earned a positive international reputation as perhaps the world's premiere expert in using THC-laden cannabis oil for effectively treating cancer and many other ailments.

Scientific experts at the revolutionary Constance Pure Botanical Extracts Company give patient-members hoping to benefit from cannabis oil access to a unique testing procedure; this protocol analyzes the sensitivity of an individual patient's cells.

The tests are done via California oncology labs. Depending on the outcome of test results, these patients sometimes become candidates to potentially undergo her increasingly popular treatments sometimes called "cannabis therapeutics."

Lab technicians use petri dishes when checking tumors to determine the most effective ratio of THC and CBD for the patient, according to an article Finley wrote for a 2015 edition of "Integrated Health Magazine." Her company has been filing patents for the technology.

"The herbal neutraceutical revolution is informed by cannabis, which is possibly the most broadly helpful plant for all mammals," Finley wrote. "Young scientists on my team work with my ideas and are starting to develop life-enhancing products that will seriously improve health, beauty and relaxation."

Finley Made Great Discoveries

While her well-deserved positive reputation spreads, Finley deserves much of the credit for positively advancing cannabis therapeutics; in the process she has made significant discoveries that some observers believe are likely to help patients suffering from various types of illness--particularly cancer.

Rather than merely calling psychoactive hemp "marijuana," Finley seems to prefer the term "cannabis." Blessed with a pleasant personality spiced with a keen intelligence, she says that cannabis use is no longer dominated by young men.

She insists that cannabis has emerged from its former status of irrelevance, prohibition and secretiveness. Instead, Finley says, science has come to the world of cannabis--thereby giving humanity the helping hand that Mother Nature always intended.

Despite these positive developments, she says that some journalists incorrectly strive to portray cannabis as a new-fangled plant. From Finley's perspective such critics incorrectly believe that the drug is quickly being legalized, faster than the necessary scientific research that normally would be needed to justify such transitions.

Rather than embracing such a "fear sells" approach used by some reporters, she correctly contends that many other countries have been much more open-minded than the United States about the issue. Those nations have extensively tested the drug.

Finley Serves a Positive Role

As her positive reputation spreads, Finley serves an increasingly important role in giving the public essential details regarding the healthful medicinal effects of cannabis.

According to the "Medical Jane" publication that specializes in marijuana news, as a San Francisco Bay Area resident, Finley was diagnosed with chronic arthritis of the sacroiliac joints and the spine--a condition called "ankylosing spondylitis." Dangerous Big Pharma drugs prescribed for the ailment almost killed her by causing a severe reaction.

Rather than continuing to suffer needlessly, Finley took positive action by reviewing studies indicating that cannabis has a positive impact on arthritis.

Blessed with boundless curiosity, intelligence and a "can-do" attitude, she then enrolled in the Oaksterdam University; the institution gives extensive instruction on cannabis--everything from cooking to medicinal uses. The university's Website describes the school as the "nation's only recognized cannabis college."

Finley then used her newfound knowledge to harvest and create a unique cannabis crop, generating extracts specifically designed to address her ailment.

The entrepreneur was "reluctant to tell her doctor that her noticeably improved health was due to cannabis," the "Medical Jane" article said. "Nonetheless, the word got out and an unnamed oncologist referred 26 Stage IV cancer patients to her for treatment. According to Finley, her cannabis oil helped treat the cancer and all but one (96 percent) of the patients remain alive."

Positive Results for Finley's Patients

Rather than using hype, Finley's professional-looking and highly informative Website gives positive, matter-of-fact details that essentially "speak for themselves."

One of the most prominent physicians quoted on the site, CBDFarm.org, is Dwight McKee, M.D., C.N.S., ABIHM, a Diplomate American Boards of Medical Oncology and Hematology.

"I've been aware of and interested in cannabis extracts for 40 years," McKee's statement on Finley's company Website says. "As an oncologist, I began recommending cannabis to cancer patients for palliation of nausea, pain and anorexia after Proposition 215 was passed in California.

"I had heard anecdotes of occasional major tumor responses of cancer patients over the years, but it wasn't until I met Constance and began to interview her patients that I saw these on a regular basis. Cannabis extracts of the proper type and amount, appear to be one of the most useful botanical medicines in supporting cancer patients."

Finley's company Website says that the firm complies

97

with regulations adopted when Golden State voters approved Proposition 215. That historic vote in the 1990s made California the first state to approve and legalize medical cannabis.

While compliant with that state's "medical cannabis collective" rules, the Constance Pure Botanical Extracts company provides cannabinoids including "artisan cannabis extracts rich in both CBD and THC."

Variety Serves as "The Spice of Life"
Striving to give patients the best possible results, Finley's company uses a variety of cannabis strains with varying potency levels. These are given only to qualified people who have become patient-members of the business's collective.

Finley's extracts company has been recommended by many physicians, thanks in large part to a good track record and attention to patients; besides oncology, the doctors' specialties include neurology, and rheumatology.

Perhaps of equal importance is the fact that, as stated by the Website, the company's cannabis oil "is intended for use as a potent medicine, not an intoxicant."

The site also indicates that cannabis oil from her company has been used as treatment for brain cancer and other forms of the disease.

Finley's Many Admirable Achievements
By many accounts, Finley has lived an amazing life embossed with numerous remarkable, admirable and noteworthy achievements.

Besides earning a master's degree in clinical psychology, she has completed intense graduate work in accounting, finance and taxation. Finley's work as a clinical psychologist proved just as successful as her career managing funds for wealthy individuals.

With equal passion, intelligence and creativity, Finley also helped provide the working poor with low-income housing--made possible by her decision to form a company that pioneered the use of tax credits.

Finley's many non-medical accomplishments deserve prominent mention, partly because her various achievements show that people passionate about achieving success also can legally and ethically help society benefit from the growing cannabis industry.

Besides creating much-needed jobs for people entering the marijuana business, Finley has played a significant and admirable role in helping to drive this new economic sector forward in a positive manner.

Overcoming Personal Hurdles

Amid Finley's previously mentioned health issues, she had become housebound for a 10-year period; she suffered from an undiagnosed autoimmune disorder. That's when the prescription drug nearly killed her.

She remembers initially being skeptical about the possibility that cannabis might relieve her symptoms; at that point she felt "prejudiced" against using the drug.

Yet Finley finally decided to try this natural remedy; she had gradually become more open-minded about the issue upon discovering cannabis treatment success stories.

Smoking cannabis controlled her pain and insomnia. Although highly motivated and energized as her health improved, Finley started worrying about the potential side effects that she might experience from regularly smoking this natural substance.

Later, while attending Oaksterdam to learn more about the drug, Finley became aware that other students apparently believed that she was a narcotics agent. Such an assumption on their part might have seemed "logical," because--after all--as her Website freely admits, "she didn't fit the mold of the typical marijuana grower or enthusiast."

Finley soon made her own cannabis oil, using instructions found on the Internet. Until then smoking the drug had only given this determined woman incremental improvement or control of her pain. The oil generated vastly superior results, changing her life for the better thanks to much more formidable pain and symptom relief.

Fully aware of the "big picture," rather than merely concentrating on herself, Finley then became increasingly determined to perfect her cannabis oil-making process in order to maximize medicinal benefits for people and other animals.

Finley Made a Milestone Achievement

To that point, Rick Simpson, an entrepreneur from Canada, had earned somewhat of a positive reputation for making and using cannabis oil, primarily for addressing cancer.

Such treatments using "Simpson oil" typically last several months, the regimens often ending when patients go into remission. (Simpson's achievements became noteworthy in their own right, as explained more fully later in this chapter.)

Cannabis oil must be free of impurities and toxic substances when used for people with medical conditions such as Finley's. Unlike cancer patients who usually take the oil for limited periods, individuals with autoimmune disorders or certain other ailments might need the substance for the remainder of their lives.

Worsening matters, Finley considered the oil's taste as "horrible" when sampling such substances provided by other cannabis collectives; those entrepreneurial ventures had created the oil by using preparation methods found online. As if this were not already enough to cause worry, she also discovered that those concoctions contained undesirable impurities and toxins.

Finley's concerns heightened even more upon realizing that the preparation methods described online for cannabis oil, typically found at the time, had never been intended for long-term ingestion. To that point, rather than eating cannabis oil the way that cancer patients need to do, recreational users typically got high on this form of the substance by smoking or inhaling vapors.

Positive Action Taken

Finley realized that patients with conditions such as hers faced the potential of long-term health problems if taking impure forms of the oil.

Determined to solve the problem, she began a five-year quest costing hundreds of thousands of dollars to purify the oil to safe levels.

The arduous, admirable and noteworthy effort proved fruitful upon the creation of her toxin-free "Constance Pure Botanical Extracts." From that point forward the respect and admiration for Finley strengthened and spread.

Her unique cannabis harvesting, manufacturing and processing protocol gained a well-deserved positive reputation for having a "pure product made with sustainably and lovingly grown, a whole plant medicine."

Thanks to Finley's dogged persistence and never-quit attitude, coupled with the effectiveness of her product, she now receives hundreds of cancer patient referrals from integrative medical oncologists.

Finley's Popularity Surged

Business accelerated at Finley's company at an increasingly rapid pace in April 2013 when a magazine published by a San Francisco Bay Area newspaper featured a positive cover story about this businesswoman and her company.

She remembers that an "overwhelming" number of desperate patients began calling for help. Determined to assist as much as possible, Finley invited a doctor of molecular biology onto her company's board.

The firm's product, customer service and efficiency soon improved even more upon setting stringent guidelines for manufacturing the oil, and cooperating with other cannabis harvesters. She worked with these growers in forming a farmer-to-patient collective, while also applying for federal patents for the company's unique oil manufacturing protocol.

Meantime, extensive research into Finley's oil is now being conducted by two different groups of doctors. Still sold for medical purposes only, never for recreational use, the product is being studied--or scheduled for future research--at:

Santa Rosa: An integrated medical practice is conducting a 50-patient study of people with Lyme Disease, to determine the oil's effectiveness in treating the condition.

Unnamed Doctors: A group of physicians and scientists at an unnamed business and location is doing a retrospective study of "all patients" who have taken the oil.

Additionally, a major research university that has not yet been revealed has agreed to function in conjunction with the retrospective study--publishing results at a later time.

Positive Media Story

Finley got widespread recognition thanks to the aforementioned positive 2013 article in the "San Francisco Weekly;" the publication described the "unheard-of" 96-percent survival rate among Stage IV cancer patients treated with her oil.

Of 28 patient-members treated with the oil, 27 of them survived as previously mentioned. This is a remarkable result by almost any account, considering the fact that only 2 percent of people with this level of the disease survive nationwide when undergoing conventional, mainstream cancer treatment.

Nonetheless, in order to be an effective remedy, the aforementioned fact that the oil has extremely high concentrations of psychoactive THC remains a must. The product might not be for everyone as a result, according to the magazine.

"Patients start with a dose as small as a grain of rice," the "San Francisco Weekly" story said. This is done "before ramping up to a full gram per day, a hit that can leave some people woozy and dizzy--uncomfortably high." Yet the vast majority of people who eat the oil become accustomed to the substance

The cost to consumers needing the oil remains expensive by some standards, as of 2013 at least $5,500 for a two-month supply, according to the magazine.

In my view such fees are a proverbial "drop in bucket," especially when considering the fact that a human life might be saved.

Unique Manufacturing Process

' According to Finley's Website, her oil has unique features designed to produce purity and to increase the product's effectiveness. Among these attributes:

Materials: When manufacturing the oil, her company refrains from using "trim" or byproducts from cannabis; such substances are sometimes found in competing oils.

Specific plants: Finley only uses the most valuable portion of the Northern California-grown female cannabis plant."

Extractors: When extracting the essential materials, Finley's company refrains from using butane or other illegal processes.

Specific targeting: Research-driven production is only for medical purposes.

Testing: Leading laboratories test the oil for potency and purity.

Cannabis strains: The company produces extracts from multiple strains, rather than using a one-plant-fits-all approach. These plants have various potencies **are** specifically designed for individual qualified patient-members.

Finley's Essential Strategy Defined

As a super-smart businesswoman, Finley deserves credit and extensive praise throughout the medical profession for using scientific methods and research.

Amid these interregal and inter-related processes, she also has enabled her company and patients to benefit from intensive participation by treating physicians.

In order to qualify for Constance Pure Botanical Extracts, a prospective patient must first contact the company via email using the contact form at the company's Website. The company typically responds to potential patients via phone and email, also contacting the person's physician if requested.

Complying with California law, in order to receive the oil from Finley's company, a patient must first become a patient-member of the business's California collective. Each of the following state-mandated requirements must be met by the patient:

Doctor: A physician licensed in the state of California must recommend that the patient use cannabis for a health ailment; only doctors are allowed to make such recommendations. Prospective patients looking for physicians qualified to make such recommendations can visit this website: 420md.org

Identification: Prospective patients must provide a legal California ID, as the company only dispenses its product within the Golden State.

Authorization: The patient must sign a collective agreement provided by the company, in order to conform with provisions of California's Health and Safety Code.

Expert Guidance Provided

Rather than merely "hand**ing** over" these valuable products to patients, the company gives each person valuable and essential guidance as they use the extract.

During their appointments, each patient is given the specific strain, potency and dosage of cannabis oil required to treat his or her specific medical condition.

Remember that besides cancer, the company legally produces and distributes extracts designed for treatment of various specific ailments.

The company helps guide patients through the stages of illness. These people have various types of cancer or other afflictions; each ailment is typically in different stages of progression.

"We provide in-depth instructions, first when you buy our

cannabis oil," the company's Website says. "And, we are available to help guide you as needed via phone consultation throughout your time as a patient-member. Most of our patients have very little or no previous experience with cannabis, and (they) find our personal coaching to be invaluable in finding their way through this treatment."

Extensive Uses Available

Via the company's Website, current or potential patient-members have access to hundreds of scholarly articles on a wide range of medical conditions that cannabis oil has been deemed effective in treating.

Besides cancer, Alzheimer's Disease and epilepsy, the many other ailments include Lyme disease, chronic pain, rheumatism, multiple sclerosis, diabetes, anxiety orders and asthma.

Online surfers can also learn why cannabis oil is different from standard medical marijuana, plus details on how THC, CBD and other cannabinoids effectively generate positive medical treatment results on a biological level.

Meet Another "Hero"

A Canadian who has received little publicity in the mainstream U.S. media, the aforementioned Rick Simpson, has been credited with using "hemp oil" for curing cancer.

Now in his senior years, Simpson lacks big-name recognition like the little girl saved by the Charlotte's Web strain of marijuana.

Yet many people who admire Simpson claim that his THC-laden oil derivative made from "hemp" or marijuana has cured many hundreds or perhaps even thousands of people with cancer.

One of the many things that make this particularly amazing is the fact that Simpson never completed high school or received a formal "scientific education."

Streams of people insist that this man is a hero for developing his natural remedy formula, while some would like to see more evidence to prove his claim.

Despite claims by Simpson's critics that his concoction has never been scientifically proven, the Internet is loaded with testimonials from cancer patients and their families--all heaping praise on him.

Process Remains Illegal

The production, possession and use of what Simpson calls "hemp oil" remains highly illegal in the United States and Canada.

According to a 2013 article in "High Times" magazine, the product Simpson produces is actually made from THC-laden hash or cannabis oil.

When produced by Simpson, according to "High Times," the oil is from cannabis indica plants--but not from pure hemp, which lacks psychoactive characteristics that famously get people "high." Simpson's concoction needs THC to be effective.

Although within the category of indica, which some people incorrectly believe always is pure "hemp," the strain preferred by Simpson is somewhat different than most marijuana that consumers typically use for getting high or for medicinal purposes.

According to various published reports, cannabis indica makes people feel "stoned" with a so-called body buzz that generates little or no impact on mental processes. This is opposed to cannabis sativa, which generates a psychoactive "high."

Besides facing a potential danger of criminal charges, people who try making their own hemp oil risk "doing it all wrong." Worsening matters, some "weed oil" products apparently are sold clandestinely using the Simpson name; the potential effectiveness of these other products not made by Simpson or Finley might seem questionable, partly because he has not endorsed or produced them.

Worsening matters, complaints have emerged, allegations by Simpson that some people have essentially ripped off his "recipe" or preparation process--before distributing the information in publications that he has never authorized.

Apparent "High-Cure" Rate

In various interviews even Simpson has admitted that not every cancer patient survives after using his natural cannabis oil remedy.

At least according to published news accounts, by Simpson's estimates a whopping average 70 percent of cancer patients survive after using his hemp oil.

This is an amazingly high cure-rate by almost any scientific standard. Only slightly more than two out of every 100 advanced Stage IV cancer patients survive in the United States when treated with standard, highly toxic chemotherapy treatments.

Simpson believes that many cancer patients who die after taking his hemp oil succumb after undergoing too much chemo, or by being physically damaged by the disease for too long. Due to these factors, he says, some patients are unable to take his creation long enough for this natural drug to improve their health.

Some people familiar with chemotherapy often say that "the chemo will kill you much faster than the cancer does."

The adverse side effects from chemo typically include nausea and vomiting, symptoms famously addressed by smoking or eating standard marijuana products other than weed oil. Also, as previously mentioned, marijuana generates hunger called "the munchies;" this attribute serves an essential role in helping to increase the body sizes of cancer patients who previously had become frail.

Heavenly Mission Continues

Simpson obviously is not in the business of "spreading the word" about his creation merely in order to "make a quick buck and run."

Instead, he has produced his creation before giving the concoction free of charge to cancer patients. Along the way he has attracted a proverbial endless waterfall of fans who all swear that his system works--in many instances saving their lives.

The Internet is filled with a growing number of testimonials from cancer patients who claim to have survived thanks to Simpson's oil. Some of these patients claim Simpson's creation "cured them," after they had been given the tragic news from mainstream doctors who proclaimed that they had less than one month to live.

Despite his milestone, earth-shattering achievements worthy of international praise, Simpson has experienced significant setbacks as a result of this charitable work; he was arrested and convicted in Canada on felony charges related to cannabis cultivation. Authorities alleged that he illegally grew cannabis, created the weed oil and unlawfully distributed those products.

Adding insult to injury, the Canadian court refused to allow testimony from the many dozens of former cancer patients who wanted to testify in Simpson's defense.

"I had people cured of cancer sitting in the court waiting to testify--they wouldn't let them on the stand!" Simpson told "High Times" magazine. "They wouldn't let me introduce any scientific evidence."

Courageous Courtroom Drama Ensued

Rather than bow to the political whims of Canadian authorities, Simpson made the difficult decision of personally defending himself in court.

While cross-examining a police official, Simpson held up a full-page newspaper article published the previous year. The story described how he helped cancer patients.

Simpson also brought definitions of the law into question when cross-examining a prosecution expert regarding the definitions of "marijuana" and "Indian hemp."

Yet a jury convicted him after only three hours deliberation, resulting in a possible 12-year jail sentence. Instead, apparently agreeing that Simpson had no criminal intent, the judge slapped him with a mere $2,000 fine without requiring probation.

This felony conviction caused another setback, the imposition of a rule blocking Simpson from traveling out of Canada. This prevents him from personally spreading the positive word about his amazing throughout the United States and in other countries.

Insult Added to Injury

Authorities piled on the damage even more, drenching the hopes of the many cancer patients worldwide who might have been able to benefit from his product.

Mirroring their reaction to the more famous Charlotte's Web marijuana strain, scientists in the United States have refrained from launching any wide-scale studies into the effectiveness of Simpson's oil.

Imagine the huge numbers of cancer patients who might be dying every day, primarily because authorities refuse to study the issue and ultimately to legalize the substance.

Unless officials change their course, society might never know whether Simpson oil works as fantastically as many people claim.

Interesting Background Details

Simpson's personal story and the oil he created seem amazing upon reviewing his somewhat humble personal background and his lack of professional medical experience. According to published reports, as a child he was bright enough to get by in class without studying a single schoolbook.

After dropping out of high school, he worked for two years at steel mills in Ontario, Canada--before returning at age 18 to his hometown, Spring Hill, Nova Scotia.

Simpson got a maintenance job at a hospital in that community during his late teens, about the time that one of his first cousins developed severe cancer. That relative died at age 22 in 1972, suffering an excruciatingly painful demise after wasting away to what medical novices call "mere skin and bones."

In numerous interviews Simpson has said that in the mid-1970s he heard a news report via car radio, unaware at the time that the report would eventually change his life and those of many others. Vaguely recalling the news report many years later, he finally developed his famed oil, initially thinking of his creation as a potential cancer cure.

Aired about two years after the death of Simpson's cousin, the broadcast chronicled how scientists at the Medical College of Virginia had used the psychoactive THC element of marijuana to kill brain tumors in laboratory mice.

Ironically, scientists had made this discovery by accident. In research for the U.S. National Institutes of Health, the scientists had been trying to prove that marijuana damages the immune system.

Curiosity Proved Beneficial

Luckily from the viewpoint of the many cancer patients who claim to have benefited from Simpson oil, he still remembered the story 23 years after that 1974 broadcast.

Everything eventually leading to his "miracle cure" evolved at a rapid-fire pace beginning in 1997. That's when Simpson suffered injuries at the hospital where he worked, caused from an aerosol spray as he put duct tape on boiler pipes that had previously been covered with asbestos.

Years later Simpson told interviewers that he inadvertently inhaled fumes from the spray that cause his body's central nervous system to temporarily stop functioning.

He instantly fell from a ladder, his head smashing against steel, a horrific smash to the skull that apparently left him unconscious for an unknown period.

Nearly 50 years old then, Simpson awakened--but had extreme

difficulty walking alone back his office. There, he remained too disoriented or physically injured to dial a telephone. Another hospital employee soon found Simpson and took him to the emergency room.

Physical Symptoms Worsened

Unable to get Simpson to remember his name, hospital personnel rushed him to a trauma center in the same building, where medical experts quickly put him on oxygen.

The extensive injury to Simpson's nervous system caused him to have jerky motions, plus headaches so severe that his head continually felt as if about to explode.

Simpson remembers that the hospital's personnel told him to go home after treating him for only three hours. Although feeling woozy, following only a few days rest he returned on Christmas Eve for his next scheduled shift.

While Simpson worked late that night the ringing in his head became louder, so severe that medical experts readmitted him to the emergency room during the wee hours of the next morning.

Simpson's perception of imagined sounds became so loud that he literally wanted to shoot himself. The noise seemed about as loud as a gas-powered lawn mower going full-bore inside a living room. Emergency room personnel also needed to quickly administer medication to control a sudden change in his blood pressure.

The following year, Simpson had to take dangerous drugs to control his ongoing symptoms caused by the accident,. Due to the medication, he often had extreme difficulty speaking an entire sentence. His ability to remember things deteriorated, so severe that reading became impossible.

Another Important Marijuana Story

In what Simpson's many loyal fans might call "somewhat of a miracle," during this period of extreme suffering he watched a TV program detailing the tremendous potential of medicinal marijuana. That episode hosted by Doctor David Suzuki was part of "The Nature of Things."

Encouraged by the report, Simpson asked his doctor if marijuana might help. But he merely got the typical type of response that many mainstream physicians still recite. The doctor told him that smoking marijuana causes lung cancer, and that researchers still needed to study cannabis before authorities could allow such prescriptions.

The physician refused to prescribe or formally recommend marijuana for Simpson. Unable to find an effective natural remedy for his condition, by 2001 he became a "chemical-zombie" due to the extremely dangerous mainstream drugs used to control his continuous and severe symptoms still caused by the 1997 injuries.

Simpson recalled that just a few months after asking his doctor about the medical marijuana, the physician told him that all available legal methods had been tried for addressing his ongoing symptoms.

Simpson's Experimentation Began

Left with no additional viable options from mainstream medicine and still recalling the news report from 23 years earlier, Simpson then began exploring the likelihood of benefiting from THC.

Believing that mainstream medicine had essentially given up on him, Simpson started taking hemp oil as his only treatment. He simultaneously stopped taking the worthless, health-wrecking traditional drugs that had exacerbated his health problems.

He soon lost weight and looked significantly younger, as the cannabis oil controlled his blood pressure, blocked his pain and finally enabled him to sleep.

Meantime, in 2003 a doctor told Simpson that spots on his skin--two on the face and one on the chest--apparently were skin cancer. The doctor removed one of them.

While the site of that initial procedure healed, Simpson experimented by placing hemp oil on bandages, which he then affixed to his remaining skin spots; they appeared to him as if red and infected, with pus oozing out.

Intrigued, he kept the bandages on his remaining spots, which the doctor likely would have needed to remove several days later.

To Simpson's amazement the two remaining skin spots had disappeared before he removed the bandages himself.

Alternative Medicine Worked Better

But then an unwanted development occurred.

A new spot appeared at the bodily site where the doctor had earlier removed a similar-looking object. This time Simpson treated himself by putting another bandage containing hemp oil atop the skin where a new spot had just reappeared.

To his delight the new red spot disappeared after just four days of self-treatment with weed oil.

Simpson visited that physician's office, eager to share these details with the doctor who had resisted the use of cannabis as treatment. Upon entering the facility, he told a receptionist--who also was the doctor's wife--about treating himself with hemp oil.

From Simpson's perspective the woman promptly went "ballistic." He remembers her exclaiming that the doctor refuses to discuss the topic and never prescribes the drug.

Simpson admits in a video available for free viewing online that this made him feel as if in "the Twilight Zone;" he perceived her response as "freaky."

Perseverance was the Key

Undaunted by the receptionist's reaction, Simpson soon applied hemp oil to the skin of his own mother. She had suffered from "weeping psoriasis," which infects skin with sores and scales. His mom's arms had become infected.

Simpson told interviewers that much to her delight, the hemp oil removed the sores and scales while stopping infection.

These significant developments marked the beginning of Simpson's persistent journey of using hemp oil to treat serious ailments--particularly cancer.

Simpson recalled that during the first year after helping himself and his mother, he successfully treated up to 60 people for their adverse skin conditions.

The following year he finally treated a man who had a "nasty looking" melanoma on his cheekbone. The man's facial cancer had previously been removed five times by licensed medical professionals, before growing back each time.

The wound completely healed during only three weeks of hemp oil treatments provided by Simpson. Apparently pleased with these results, the man also suffered from glaucoma, a severe eye disease causing blindness unless successfully treated.

To treat glaucoma mainstream physicians often prescribe eyedrops produced by major pharmaceutical companies. Yet the eyedrops and even operations using lasers and tubes occasionally fail to relieve intraocular pressure, thereby resulting in blindness.

The man started eating weed oil, becoming the first person that Simpson treated this way other than himself. The man's intraocular pressure lowered to helpful levels, perhaps saving his eyesight.

Helping Services Spread

Encouraged by these results, Simpson started giving hemp oil to other people, particularly several individuals suffering from internal cancer.

While Simpson had become increasingly confident about his hemp oil's healing powers, at this stage he provided this natural substance to a woman who had been told by physicians she had only weeks to live after a Stage IV cancer diagnosis.

Upon taking Simpson's oil, the woman's cancer disappeared and she regained good health.

According to Simpson, around that time his oil also started curing diabetes, relieving people of insulin dependence.

To steadily build resistance to the oil, patients initially eat extremely small amounts before gradually building their intake. According to "High Times," eating one gram daily "can be disorienting, but many adapt rapidly to the pharmacological effects."

Authorities Tightened the Noose

To this point for the most part Simpson had readily given his oil to people suffering from health problems after they learned about him via word-of-mouth.

Yet his so-called "low-level operation" inadvertently got unwanted publicity that eventually led to his previously mentioned arrest.

Authorities learned of Simpson's cannabis-related activities after he started treating people at a local chapter of the Royal Canadian Legion. At least one person there had unsuccessfully tried to convince authorities that the oil was effectively "curing" many people. The Legion member urged the officials to pay positive attention, so that they hopefully could learn more about this sensational remedy--in order to eventually enable far more people to benefit.

Rather than take a positive stance, however, authorities responded by arresting Simpson under the criminal charges that he eventually was convicted of committing.

At this point one of Simpson's acquaintances had started giving the oil to a man dying of advanced Stage IV lung cancer. This patient's condition supposedly improved, and he was taken by ambulance from the hospital to his home. His lungs cleared.

Encouraged by these results, a relative of this patient scheduled a meeting at the Legion Hall, where he hoped officials would review evidence and then reach their own conclusions.

Instead, officials changed the locks on the Hall's doors to prevent the meeting.

Positive Action Continues

Following his conviction, Simpson took a positive and courageous stand on the issue. Instead of "caving in" to the destructive preferences of authorities and the draconian marijuana laws, he aggressively continued efforts to teach the general public about the oil's many positive medical benefits.

With producer Christian Laurette, he made the "Run from the Cure" video available for viewing for free on the Internet. In this instance, the word "cure" refers to standard chemotherapy, which might kill more people than the cancers.

The compelling video brought the positive news regarding cannabis oil to many thousands of people, most who had never previously known about the treatment.

Some cancer patients admittedly had been skeptical prior to viewing the film. But intrigued after watching the video, many eventually started taking the oil as a natural treatment. Lots of them insist that the oil works, particularly when used by cancer patients who have not previously been treated with chemotherapy.

Yet the multibillion-dollar pharmaceutical industry--plus the many doctors and medical complexes--are unlikely to ever approve of the oil as a viable and preferable treatment. Such a change would threaten the physicians' monopoly of using only Big Pharma-approved drugs.

Sadly, this prohibition denies many cancer patients of an apparent cure.

Even Simpson has stated in numerous interviews and on videos featuring him that major pharmaceutical companies are unlikely to give up their lucrative corner of the cancer-treatment market--"no matter how many dead bodies pile up."

Positive Evidence Accumulated

Recent scientific research in other nations has proven this remedy is effective in treating cancer, despite the combined efforts of authorities in Canada and the United States to block reliable research into Simpson's oil and medicinal marijuana.

According to news media reports, researchers in Spain successfully used THC to remove fast-moving brain cancer in two human patients. Scientists believe that this unique substance causes "autophagy," a biological process in which cancer cells self-destruct by essentially "feeding on themselves." (See Chapter X.)

Sadly, however, the mainstream liberal U.S. news media has never broadly mentioned significant findings such as these. North American journalists seem to show "blind faith," fully trusting corrupt or inept government bureaucracies.

Once again, the big losers here are everyday consumers and patients suffering from a variety of adverse health conditions and diseases--particularly cancer.

Meantime, the media still has the time and resources to report on the occasional arrests of people who provide cannabis oil to people suffering from the disease.

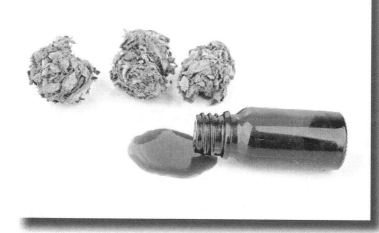

13

Streams of Positive Comments About "Cannabis Oil"

On a consistent basis the Internet is being filled with positive comments about the product that Simpson prefers for a variety of reasons to call "hemp oil," although it primarily consists of THC-laden materials from flowering female cannabis indica plants. (Remember, as previously stated, many people mistakenly believe that if a plant has indica characteristics it is "hemp" that fails to generate a high; this is untrue because many plants containing indica characteristics are still psychoactive. In order to be classified as pure "hemp," a plant must have an extremely low THC content--far below 1 percent. By contrast, Simpson's concoction reportedly has a THC level of nearly 68 percent.)

Images and statements from free YouTube videos can be rebroadcast on the Internet or published elsewhere. In order to post their videos for free viewing on YouTube, the owners must first acknowledge that the videos are not copyrighted. Then, upon uploading the video to the YouTube Website, the film then becomes part of the "public domain."

A review of a handful of statements from Simpson-related films on YouTube reveal lots of positive but highly emotional comments. Lots of these statements are given from the hearts of the appreciative people involved. Here is just a brief sampling of some of these comments, edited for brevity:

Simpson: To anyone that would say that I'm nothing but a high-class drug dealer, to that I would just have to laugh. Drug dealers, they sell it for a big price and then they make the money. (Unlike them), I've been giving it away since 2003. Now, I'd have to be the stupidest drug dealer in history to give it away, now wouldn't I?

I'm just trying to help people. I mean, that's all that this is about. And I want people to know how to heal themselves.

Officials: At one point Simpson contacted the Canadian Cancer Society to tell them that he had identified his oil as an effective cure. According to a posting by Simpson in an online video, the organization responded by saying: "The Society does not support or endorse medical products or dietary supplements. Thanks for the information. We wish you luck in your work."

Professional report: According to a report posted on one of the videos, the "Lancet Medical Journal" stated that: "Chemotherapy kills more people than it saves."

Simpson: The government and the medical system do not want you to have the ability to cure your own diseases. These people don't want anything to change. They've got the big cars; they've got the big bank accounts ... They don't give a damn about the poor people.

Man No. 1: There seems to be a lot of things that this can help. And it's just a sin that we're not allowed to find out more, for the sake of the ungodly dollar. I mean that's what it boils down to, right? I mean people should have a right in this country to keep themselves well--that should be a basic right. I thought it was supposed to be that, but I'm finding out 'not so much.'

Man No. 2: (After telling a doctor that he was using THC-laden oil to treat illness, the doctor) froze right in his tracks. I told him a story that I heard that it would work. And I said, "Will it work, or will it not?" Now, he (the doctor) said, "to be honest about it, I cannot confirm it, and I cannot deny it."

Man No. 3: There are so many people out there suffering, with so many diseases that this works for. And at night I don't sleep very well, because I think of those little children that are being poisoned, and that are being fed chemotherapy and radiation ... This is so horrible.

Man No. 2: Find out how good it is. Well, I know it's good. But listen, it's (also) more than just good for cancer.

Simpson: If you have a serious medical condition such as cancer, what right does anyone have to tell you that you cannot use hemp medicine?

Man No. 4: Take a look at me six months ago (while suffering from cancer). I was up and down, and I had no energy with nothing to do. But right now (after being treated with Simpson's oil), I want to live. ... God put it out there for us. Why aren't we using it? Why are we denying (Simpson) this (ability to distribute the oil), somebody that's going to save someone else's life?

Simpson: If people would just realize how much this medicine can help them, the world would be a better place.

Man No. 2: It's a miracle medicine. There is no way around that. ... In January 2007, my father came to live with my wife and I because at this point his cancer had become unmanageable and he could not stay alone anymore. He had fluid in both of his lungs and could not even hardly walk around. His breathing had gone down to 70 percent, and he was on his last legs. We started him on the treatment, and inside of three months the cancer was completely gone and in between that he got nothing but better. The man improved every day from the time that he started the oil.

Man No. 2: Change your life. Take some real medicine-- medicine that is safe, and medicine that works for a change.

Simpson: (The plant used to make the oil cannot be patented because it's a natural substances. Thus to drug companies, this means) no money. ... This oil has brought many people right off of their death beds. But due to the many restrictions put in place by our government against this medicine, we feel that it is our duty to inform the public how they can make their own.

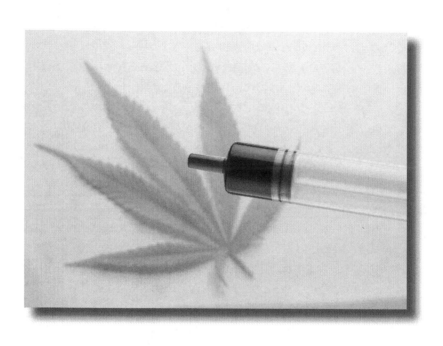

14

How to Make "Cannabis Oil"

Producing oil derived from cannabis involves an extremely dangerous process.

The complexity of this challenge becomes even more formidable when considering the fact that making the oil is highly illegal in the United States and Canada.

Any person or group of people must realize that when trying to make the oil they do so at their own risk, both from injury and also the possibility of arrest and conviction.

In order to effectively treat cancer or other ailments, as previously stated the oil must contain at least some of the psychoactive ingredient called THC.

Worsening matters, some unscrupulous marijuana distributors apparently produce hemp oil containing contaminants or lacking THC needed for treatments to be effective. For this reason, some experienced users of medicinal cannabis and recreational marijuana strongly recommend that consumers avoid purchasing this oil "on the street."

Additionally, consumers should be wary of any product sold online labeled as "Simpson oil." Most of the time consumers have no way of knowing whether such products have been endorsed by him, or if they contain the necessary medicinal attributes-- especially THC.

As if these issues were not already enough to cause extreme concern, Simpson has complained that in at least one instance someone allegedly has used his data in publishing other books that supposedly describe specifics of the unique process that he personally developed.

Due to all of these challenging factors, people considering whether to attempt to make the oil on their own should first study all of their city, state or national regulations involving marijuana.

Ultimately, anyone who decides to produce the oil must realize that they are "doing so at their own risk. You are fully responsible for the decisions that you make, and no one is asking you to do this or recommending that you do it."

Simpson Has Detractors

Whether out of jealousy, ignorance or genuine concern, some people complain or have personal reservations about Simpson and his increasingly famous oil. Among issues they cite:

Knowledge: From his critics' perspective, Simpson lacks medical training that would be needed to cure cancer.

Licensing: No one seems to accuse or imply that Simpson is practicing medicine without a license. And he has never proclaimed to be a physician and never behaves like such a person. Yet critics contend that anyone who "goes around trying to cure cancer" should have a medical license.

Proof: At least from his critics' perspective, Simpson supposedly lacks proof of his claim that an average of 70 percent of cancer patients who eat the oil are cured of the disease.

Research: There have been no focused scientific studies to prove the oil's apparent effectiveness in killing cancer. There also has never been extensive research into any apparent long-term health effects experienced by current or former cancer patients who have eaten hemp oil.

Simpson Has Supporters

As briefly mentioned earlier, Simpson also has streams of fans. Among the most famous is entertainer Tommy Chong of "Cheech and Chong," a 1970s comic duo famous for their irreverent humor that involved the smoking of marijuana.

A native Canadian, now a naturalized U.S. citizen born in 1938, Chong announced in June 2012 that he was suffering from prostate cancer. Just one month later Chong revealed on CNN that he was "99-percent cancer free" after taking Simpson oil, in conjunction with a modified diet.

Chong said that he was "drug-free" during the three years immediately before being diagnosed with cancer. Circumstances prevented him from using marijuana while incarcerated, following a felony conviction for financing a company that distributed bongs used to smoke marijuana. Federal law enforcement officers had arrested Chong after targeting companies that illegally sold drug paraphernalia online.

At least for Chong, many years of using cannabis had failed to prevent the development of cancer. Yet he said that the specific use of highly concentrated cannabis oil apparently "did the trick" in eliminating his cancer.

Understand Basic Terminology

Remember, as previously stated, Simpson prefers to call his creation "hemp oil," although the substance is not derived from pure hemp--which lacks high-level therapeutic amounts of THC.

Actually, standard marijuana contains high levels of THC, while hemp has only minuscule amounts of this psychoactive substance. This hails as the primary factor differentiating marijuana from hemp. The oil must have ample THC levels in order tgo be effective. A full 100-percent "hemp-only strain" falls in the category of cannabis sativa, used for a wide range of industrial products, and foods.

A major online encyclopedia describes hemp this way: "*Cannabis sativa* L. Subs. *Sativa* var. *Sativa* is the variety grown for industrial use, while C. *Sativa* subs. *Indica* generally has poor fiber quality and is primarily used for recreational and medical purposes."

Cannabis sativa is categorized within the cannabis genus, a subspecies that biologists call part of the "Cannabaceae family."

According to "High Times," for making his oil, Simpson prefers to use cannabis indica plants, which biologists do not consider as "hemp."

In order to be legally classified as permissible "hemp" in Canada, a plant must have a measurable THC level of less than one-third of a percent (0.3 percent).

By comparison, most marijuana used today for medicinal and recreational purposes have average THC levels from 18 percent to 25 percent.

Basic Production Procedures

People should use extreme caution when following so-called recipes for the oil. So, refrain from using any preparation method found online or in print that lacks Simpson's official endorsement.

Although Simpson is not a doctor and he lacks in-depth scientific education in the medical field, he apparently has developed specific processes for preparing, storing, shipping and using the oil that famously has his surname.

As a result, you will not find his specific "recipe" here. The only place to find and purchase Simpson's recommendations in print form is via his Website--PhoenixTears.ca.

Please note that the designation or address for his site is not a dot-com. Instead, his Website uses a "CA" country code, a term that specifies that his Website originates in Canada. So, when attempting to visit the site, refrain from typing in dot-com. Instead, with no blank spaces immediately after writing PhoenixTears in your Web browser, type a period immediately followed by the letters "CA."

Simpson's 199-page book, "Phoenix Tears, Rick Simpson Oil ~ Nature's Answer for Cancer," is available in eBook form via Amazon.com.

From his Web page, consumers can purchase an eBook version of his two publications, apparently available in a .PDF format. One features his life story, while the other gives specifics on his methods for producing and using the oil.

Basics About Preparation

While the in-depth written specifics about Simpson's production methods are only available from his publications, he has discussed generalities regarding this system in videos seen for free on YouTube. As previously stated, any comments posted on that online service become part of the public domain, meaning that those statements can be repeated or redistributed.

So a summary of those general comments is shown below, provided here as a convenience for anyone who later chooses to get more specific details via his Website.

At least one of the videos with a voice-over by Simpson features this written message: "Making your own oil is extremely dangerous and we do not approve of this method." This disclaimer makes clear that people who attempt to produce weed oil on their own should realize that they would be doing so at their own risk.

After this introduction, Simpson's voice is heard as he describes the production process, while the video shows rotating images of cannabis and oil-filled pots.

"Sativa strains produce an oil that is a very good anti-depressant and tends to energize a person, while most of the oil that I produce come from indica strains.

"Indica strains tend to relax a person and give them more sleep. Rest and sleep are part of the healing process."

After stating this, for nearly 2 minutes and 30 seconds Simpson describes the step-by-step process:

Container: Place the starting material, preferably good bud, in a plastic container.

Moisture: Dampen the material inside the container with the solvent that you are using. (Specifics of the solvent are not described in the video; consumers apparently must get details about the solvent from his publications.)

Crushing: After adding the solvent, crush the bud material. (Simpson is shown pushing a wood stick into the cannabis. The video does not explain how long this should be done, or specifics on how to effectively crush the material.)

More solvent: After fully crushing the material, add more solvent until the cannabis is completely covered. (The amount of solvent is not fully described in the video.) He mentions isopropyl alcohol as one of the possible solvents.

Continue: Work and stir for at least three minutes to allow the THC to dissolve into the solvent.

Strain: Drain the solvent from the material, using a coffee filter.

Appearance change: The solvent now resembles the color of gasoline, due to the presence of hemp oil.

Essential ventilation: For safety reasons, make sure that the area where this mixing, filtering and boiling off of solvents happens is well-ventilated, in order to safely and effectively remove harmful fumes that might otherwise cause injury. The idea is to remove the fumes in order to reduce the danger of an explosion or fire.

Use Special Care: Take precautions to ensure that the fumes never contact red-hot elements or a spark; doing so could ignite the fumes from the solvent. (A no-smoking sign is shown.)

Container: Simpson has found that an electric rice cooker is useful for effectively boiling off the solvent.

Temperature: Bring the solvent-oil mix in the rice cooker to a boil.

Ventilation: Use a fan to carry away the fumes from the solvent.

More fluid: As the solvent boils off, continue adding more solvent-oil mix until it is done.

Add water: Add eight to 10 drops of water as the level in the boiling pot comes down for the last time. Since the boiling point of water is much higher than the boiling point of the solvent, the water allows the solvent to be released as the oil thickens.

Final processes: As the final solvent is being released, it's a good idea to lift the rice cooker, and keep the contents in the cooker moving. (Hands are shown holding the pot, while gently swirling the hot materials still inside the cooker.) Keep the contents of the cooker moving. This helps to release any remaining solvent, and also protects the oil from too much heat. At no time should the temperature of the oil exceed 290 degrees Fahrenheit.

Container: Gently pour the oil from the rice cooker into a small metal container.

Dehydration: Put the container that holds the oil into a dehydrator, or put the container on a gentle-heating device such as a coffee warmer. A few hours may be needed to evaporate the water off the oil.

Result: In the end, there should be no bubbling or other activity on the surface of the oil, which becomes quite runny when hot. But when cooled it takes on the consistency of a thick grease. Generally, a pound of good hemp bud will produce about two ounces of high-grade oil.

Cure: Ingesting two ounces of high-grade oil over a two month to three month period is enough to cure most cancers, Simpson said.

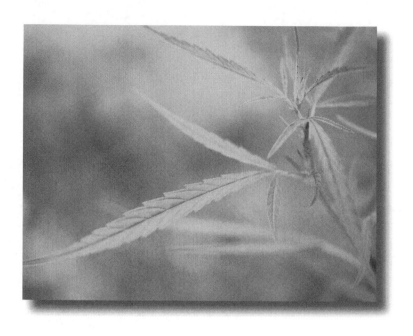

15

Discover What Generates That "High"

Although just one of the 483 compounds found in a single marijuana plant, THC acts as the primary psychoactive ingredient that makes users "high."

Labeled with the scientific name of "tetrahydrocannabinol," this serves as the primary ingredient that many users actively want for "getting stoned."

Typical symptoms include a mild or even intense euphoria, accompanied by a heightened mood and occasionally nagging hunger called "the munchies."

The yearning to get high usually serves as the top motivating factor for most users, primarily as a stress reducer--although some people experience paranoia or anxiety as the result of THC.

As previously stated, scientists in Israel became the first researchers to identify THC in 1964. Until then marijuana had spread worldwide in gradual phases over thousands of years, without people knowing exactly how or what within marijuana plants made them high.

Consider Rose Bush Thorns

THC serves as nature's way of protecting the marijuana plant, similar at least in some sense to the way that thorns naturally help protect rose bushes.

Scientists believe that through the evolutionary process many plants including marijuana developed individualized "self-defense" mechanisms against potential predators.

Some researchers believe that THC helps to ward off "herbivores," animals including mammals or insects that might strive to eat or destroy marijuana plants.

Besides thorns, some plants produce self-defense mechanisms ranging from waxes and resins to inedible fuzzy hairlike outgrowths called "trichome."

The chemical compound within THC likely is extremely dangerous or even fatal to some natural potential predators of marijuana plants.

Protection Against Harmful Rays

According to a 1987 article in "Phytochemistry," THC likely serves as a mechanism to protect cannabis plants from potentially harmful ultraviolet rays.

Some scientists believe--or at least they have speculated--that THC prevents the absorption of dangerous rays emitted by the sun, thereby protecting the plant from potentially serious or even destructive damage.

Typical marijuana users likely remain unaware of these apparent factors. All these people really care about is getting high.

On a scientific level, THC possesses what scientists call "aromaticity," which in this case should never be confused with any unique aroma or odor.

Instead, the aromaticity of THC refers to the unusually stable nature of its atoms, formed as relatively flat rings, naturally placed in unique double-bonds that interact with each other.

Unique Atom Structures

Marijuana users essentially have "lucked out" or struck the "biological jackpot" thanks to the double-bonding of atoms within THC.

Thanks to this unique characteristic, THC retains its psychoactive properties even when burned for smoking, or cooked when putting marijuana into baked products.

However, despite these amazing abilities of THC to transform and protect itself, any of this substance directly exposed to flames automatically self-destructs. For this reason, marijuana users who prefer to smoke rather than eat the drug should only briefly use flames when lighting their cannabis.

Adding to the "benefits," at least from the perspective of marijuana users, THC also features unique "Terpenoid" characteristics.

This essentially means that besides its unique ability to retain double-bonded atoms, THC has medicinal, antibacterial and pharmaceutical attributes.

Terpenoids are abundant throughout nature, within natural substances including herbs often used by Homeopathic physicians as effective natural remedies.

Terpenoids also can be derived from common herbs. These range from cinnamon, cloves and ginger, to the red substance in tomatoes and the yellow coloring of sunflowers.

Terpenoids are found within the many cannabinoids of cannabis, and also from cannabinoids derived from ginkgolide and biobalide, each within Ginkgo biloba.

Generates Pain Relief

According to a 2001 article in "Biological Sciences," THC works as more than a psychoactive drug--but also as a mild to moderate analgesic effective for pain relief.

If this theory is correct, besides getting users "high," THC naturally fights pain like other plants or plant-based products found in nature such as willow tree bark used to make aspirin.

THC generates pain relief via interaction with dorsal root ganglion within the spinal cord, and also via "Periaqueductal gray," the body's primary pain control center.

Along with the previously mentioned appetite stimulation, the drug also impacts the body's sight, hearing and taste--while sometimes generating a feeling of fatigue.

While these symptoms might seem harmless, some users experience energy reductions or increases in aggression during withdrawal.

Unique & Helpful Characteristics

Boosting the effectiveness of THC even more, the drug actually serves as a mild antioxidant, according to a 2008 article in the "International Journal of Obesity."

This emerges as somewhat significant, largely because antioxidants destroy free radicals that might lead to cancer if left unchecked.

In chemistry, a "free radical" is an unpaired ion, molecule or atom that sometimes generates oxidative stress that sometimes results in cancer.

Despite the unique characteristic of THC as an anti-oxidant in preventing or removing free radicals, people who often get high on the drug should refrain from saying: "I'm doing this to avoid getting cancer."

Scientists lack any definitive study results indicating that cannabis prevents the disease. Yet as previously mentioned streams of consumers statements insist that when administered under specific conditions, concentrated "marijuana oil," "weed oil," or "Simpson oil" destroys cancers that would kill the person if left unchecked.

16
Undeniable Marijuana Dangers

Like all drugs including alcohol, marijuana poses some potential dangers, particularly when abused in excessive quantities.

Many people and pro-marijuana organizations in recent years have claimed that there has never been a documented case of a fatal psychoactive cannabis overdose.

While that might be true, everyone considering the use of-- or already taking--the drug should know its potential dangers or adverse effects.

For the most part, the natural substances of marijuana and THC are generally safe when consumed in low or moderate amounts.

According to a 2014 report in the "American Journal of Cardiology," numerous reports link marijuana smoking to an increased risk of heart attack.

In addition, some anti-marijuana groups contend that physicians lack adequate information on the possible toxicity of THC.

All previous studies on the potential toxic impact of this substance have been performed on animals other than humans, according to various reports.

Fatal Overdoses Unlikely

Numerous medical studies filed with the National Library of Medicine indicate that a fatal overdose from marijuana is almost impossible.

These documents indicate that in order to administer a lethal dose of marijuana a person would have to receive the intravenous equivalent of 960 capsules of THC.

From among 1,619 people treated with cannabis and THC in

clinical trials, 6.9 percent of them discontinued treatment due to adverse side effects.

Simultaneously, 2.2 percent of 1,118 people treated with placebos chose to discontinue those pills after complaining of supposedly negative symptoms.

One of the patients died during the study; the death was listed as "possibly related" to the drug. The report failed to list whether the person suffered from epilepsy.

Researchers refrained from detailing the side effects experienced by the patients. Symptoms ranged from "suicidal ideation" to hallucination.

Reliable Studies Unavailable
Reliable and unbiased studies on the long-term effects of using marijuana for an extended period have been unavailable.

Until marijuana became legalized for recreational use in four states and the District of Columbia, the drug's researchers had only one legal source--the National Institute on Drug Abuse.

Many people claim that institution has an obvious pre-ordained bias against marijuana and particularly THC. By some accounts, about 94 percent of all federally funded studies on psychoactive cannabis have focused on apparent harm caused by the drug, rather than striving to identify any benefits.

Some doctors and consumers hope for more extensive studies, as increasing numbers of states relax their anti-marijuana laws or legalize the drug.

Even without such additional research, almost all casual observers know that while high on marijuana people experience impaired cognitive abilities.

Besides difficulties in organizing and making decisions, while "high on weed" people have problems making plans due to slow mental functioning.

Until now the various scientific studies on these factors have generated mixed results. Researchers say that separate studies fail to categorize long-term users, people who infrequently used the drug, and those who have never been stoned on marijuana.

Teen Use Questioned

Families and some researchers in recent years also have insisted that much more extensive studies need to be done on marijuana's long-term health impacts on teenagers.

The brain matures throughout childhood, and particularly throughout the vital physical and mental maturation processes of a person's teens, and later as young adults into their mid-20s.

Scientists need to learn more about whether extensive cannabis use among teens adversely impacts the long-term IQ and cognitive abilities of these people during later life past age 30.

Until now all states that have legalized marijuana have done so only for adults. Many people worry that teens in those jurisdictions will think that because marijuana has been legalized for adults that "weed is OK for them."

Ultimately, the concern focuses on whether society is giving mixed messages to teenagers, essentially telling them: "You must do as I say, but not what I do myself."

Disturbing Report About Psychosis

As reported by a March 2005 article in the "Journal of Psychopharmacology," adolescents using cannabis have an increased risk of psychosis.

If true, this finding emerges as particularly disturbing, partly because the term "psychosis" scientifically describes a "loss of contact with reality."

Often described as "psychotic," such individuals experience personality changes and a condition called "thought disorder"--an inability to think in an organized manner.

A separate 2004 study concluded that although cannabis doubly increases the risk of psychosis--the drug does not necessarily cause this condition.

Even so, concern intensified in 2009 when a French study concluded that cannabis increased the probability of schizophrenic disorders, particularly if used before age 15.

Additional Concerns Emerged

Adding to the concerns, at least according to a 2007 report in "Lancet," all people using cannabis have a greater probability of developing psychosis than non-users.

A different study indicated that cannabis negatively impacts one of the body's natural and essential enzymes called "catechol-o-methyl transferase."

Often called "COMT," when healthy this enzyme positively interacts with important substances critical to optimal brain function.

A report by the "British Journal of Psychiatry" later cast doubt on the theory that that cannabis alters the vital COMT enzymes.

The overall issue got further attention in 2008 when a German report blamed cannabis as a casual factor in at least some instances of schizophrenia.

Needless to say, much more extensive study needs to be done on the possibility that cannabis generates psychosis, particularly as more governments legalize the drug.

17

World Famous High

What is it like to "get high" on marijuana?

Some people claim the best and most effective way to discover the sensation of getting stoned on cannabis is "simply to do it."

Yet to do so, even for a brief "first and only time," would emerge as the equivalent of delving into the immoral realm within the personal belief systems of some people.

Others might want to avoid the drug due to fears of harsh anti-marijuana laws, or in an effort to prevent possible personal harm after learning of potential dangers.

These various converging factors are added to the fact that many officials still proclaim cannabis as an extremely dangerous "doorway drug," supposedly leading to the abuse of dangerous narcotics.

Getting Stoned: Symptoms Vary

First-timers, so-called "amateurs," and even experienced stoners need to know that the symptoms and sensations often vary greatly when getting high.

The level of "feeling stoned" and the specific symptoms of each session can vary depending on a variety of factors. Among them:

Amounts: Smaller quantities consumed generally generate less symptoms than when smoking or eating significant amounts over limited periods of time. A cannabis plant with extremely high THC content results in an extremely intense high.

Personal history: People with an extensive personal history of getting high sometimes need more than other people in a single session to feel stoned. This occurs because the body occasionally becomes accustomed to cannabinoids, particularly as a result of persistent long-term use.

Temporary cessation: People who often use marijuana sometimes choose to occasionally abstain from the drug for extended periods, in order to naturally rid their bodies of cannabis. During this "detox period," the body becomes less accustomed to using the drug. This way people who undergo "temporary detox," hope to get "higher than ever" upon restarting to use of marijuana.

Asymptomatic: Some people report that when smoking or eating cannabis for the first time they fail to experience any sensation of getting high--perhaps because their bodies initially fail to absorb the substance. In most of these rare instances the high finally occurs in subsequent uses.

Eating verses Smoking: The high from smoking can occur almost instantly, usually lasting up to a few hours. By contrast, eating food that contains marijuana can take up to an hour or more to generate a high, sometimes lasting up to 10 hours. These differences occur because smoking instantly forces THC into the bloodstream, while the digestive process invariably takes much longer to generate the body's natural absorption of this psychoactive ingredient into the blood.

Body weight factors: People with large body masses such as extremely tall or overweight individuals often require more cannabis to get stoned, compared to people of relatively small physical stature. Conversely, people with little bodies sometimes need only small amounts to feel stoned. Overall these "big and small" factors are somewhat similar to those differences in inebriation levels among people who ingest alcohol.

Unique Symptoms Occur

Some marijuana users claim the drug causes a relatively pleasant high, a sharp contrast to alcohol--a depressant.

Beer, wine and hard liquor are depressants that often generate negative behaviors and emotions.

By contrast, many of these individuals claim that when high on marijuana they generally experience fairly pleasant, and positive sensations; users describe this as a mild or intense "euphoria."

From the view of these individuals, getting drunk only serves to make them feel more depressed about themselves and about the world in general. To them, the use and symptoms of alcohol are often centered on sadness, coupled with psychological and physiological addictions. Although alcohol is generally a depressant, while inebriated many people behave as if the most likable individuals imaginable. Still others have a tendency to become violent when drunk.

A completely opposite approach and perspective occurs with cannabis, often described as causing mild or intense happy sensations--an overall feeling of "peace." And some studies or medical reports indicate that marijuana is less addictive to the body and mind.

Without "Sweeping Generalities"

From the view of at least some scientists, these broad overall descriptions comparing the highs of cannabis and alcohol are merely "sweeping generalities."

Scientists insist that the effects of any psychoactive high from cannabis can vary significantly--often depending on the specific plant, method of use and individual person.

Ultimately, in order to give a "high," THC must first enter the bloodstream before eventually interacting and binding with cannabinoid receptors within the brain.

On a biological level, THC impacts many of the brain's vital neurotransmitters--particularly norepinephrine and dopamine, natural substances that generate mild euphoria.

Paradoxically, at least according to some scientists, these cannabinoid systems sometimes generate anxiety, rather than just euphoria.

Overall "Good" Sensations

The so-called "positive effects" most frequently mentioned regarding THC involve "good factors" that include:

Feelings of well-being: A sense that "all is right and perfect in this peaceful world," a mental sensation that nothing could possibly go wrong.

Relaxation: The mental feelings of any stress virtually disappear or significantly decrease, making the person feel free or void of any significant problems.

Happy: Many people claim the high of cannabis makes them laugh far more often than when sober, thanks to an intensified appreciation for humor.

Positive perspective: THC and cannabis overall can alter an individual's perception, often--some of them claim--"for the better."

Jovial behavior: Some cannabis users claim the drug makes them feel far more "jovial," in a happy, sharing party-oriented mood--feeling less reclusive than when sober.

Enhanced recollection: Sometimes called "episodic memory," this involves an enhanced ability to recall specific past experiences in great detail.

Increased sensuality: Partly due to the significant decrease in stress, some cannabis users feel extremely amorous when stoned--far more than usual.

Sensations: THC often generates sharply increased awareness of sensations, particularly taste, touch, smells and sounds.

Creativity: Lacking the stress that permeates their lives when sober, many cannabis users report a sharply enhanced inspiration and ability to create.

Open Thought Pathways

Perhaps best of all, at least from the perspective of some marijuana users, the drug sharply boosts their abstract thinking.

For many people, this supposedly involves a significant

improvement in their individual abilities to perceive "the overall big picture" involving their own lives.

However, while all these many supposedly positive symptoms might seem fantastic, numerous negative effects occasionally occur.

Up to 30 percent of recreational cannabis smokers experience panic attacks, anxiety, or a combination of both, according to a 2011 "Harvard Mental Health Letter."

Another frequent symptom that can be perceived as either positive or negative involves a distortion of the sense of time. This happens when the person thinks that an activity took an extremely long time, when in fact only a few minutes occurred.

Also, the previously mentioned "munchies" sometimes involve eating large quantities of food, such as an entire carton of ice cream.

Potential Mental Issues

Marijuana sometimes causes a mental disorder in which people feel as if detached from themselves, according to a 2005 report in a Hebrew publication, "Harefuah."

This potentially serious condition called "depersonalization" leaves people feeling as if having no control over situations, while seeming as mysteriously and mentally "somehow watching themselves."

To many people suffering from this disorder, everything seems as if vague or even dreamlike, seemingly as if the world lacks significance.

People who refrain from taking drugs sometimes suffer from depersonalization as a result of trauma or extreme anxiety.

Psychiatrists list depersonalization as a common symptom of various mental disorders ranging from schizophrenia to migraines and clinical depression.

Typical mainstream treatments often hinge on the underlying cause; possible remedies range from prescription drugs to psychotherapy.

Severe Symptoms Possible

Excessive marijuana use reportedly has caused severe mental problems in extremely rare cases, although well-documented instances are difficult to find.

Marijuana has caused some users of the drug to suffer acute psychosis lasting up to six hours, according to a 2012 book by Donald G. Barceloux.

However, many people seem to doubt Barceloux's claims, insisting that they have been unable to find any documented reports of such instances.

His book, "Medical Technology of Drug Abuse," says that among heavy users some of these symptoms have continued for many days.

The book subtitled "Synthesized Chemicals and Psychoactive Plants" claims that doctors need to use physical restraint and sedation when marijuana-induced psychosis causes aggression.

Marijuana's Hallucinogenic Qualities

Many doctors and scientists consider marijuana and particularly THC as a mild or moderate hallucinogen, a drug causing changes to thoughts, emotions and consciousness.

Hallucinogenics within the cannabis classification typically cause one or more mental symptoms or reactions lasting for limited periods.

These effects often involve an alteration or change in the person's perception.

Unlike dreams that typically occur in a related phenomenon while asleep, drug-induced hallucinations occur when the individual is awake.

Scientists seem to engage in an ongoing debate regarding which drugs should be listed as "psychedelic" or "hallucinogenic."

Although these terms and symptoms are sometimes intermingled, psychedelics usually are listed within a harder-class of dangerous drugs such as LSD and heroin.

Other Neurological Effects

Marijuana often negatively impacts short-term memory, according to a 1999 book, "Marijuana and Medicine: Assessing the Science Base."

The book by J.E. Joy, S.J. Watson Jr., and J.A. Benson Jr., says this occurs when cannabinoid interacts with CB1 receptors in the hippocampus area of the brain.

Besides enabling the individual to manage spatial perception, the hippocampus plays essential roles in generating short-term and long-term memories.

This essential region of the brain serves a vital role in making an active and vibrant life possible. Alzheimer's disease and other serious conditions such as oxygen depravation can severely damage the hippocampus, essentially damaging brain function.

Yet scientists apparently lack any conclusive evidence that cannabis use and THC seriously injures or harms this vital region of the brain.

Even so, scientific researchers and even casual marijuana users realize--or at least they should acknowledge--that the drug invariably blocks or hampers short-term memory.

As previously indicated, the apparent or possible long-term impact of cannabis on the hippocampus and the overall brain remains inconclusive.

Impacts on the Hippocampus

Scientists know that while high on cannabis and THC, the drug interacts with neurotransmitters within the hippocampus.

This interaction, in turn, causes a decrease in neuronal activity within this region of the brain--thereby causing the short-term memory loss.

These conclusions were chronicled in a 2006 report published in "Molecular Pharmaceutics." It lists THC as considerably superior to other drugs commonly prescribed for Alzheimer's.

According to a wide variety of news reports, in recent years scientists in various research projects have reached similar findings.

Technically, however, at least as of early 2015, lawmakers in some states including Utah had rejected efforts to allow the use of marijuana in treating the disease.

Driving While High

Various publications have listed conflicting reports on whether marijuana use adversely impacts a person's ability to safely drive motor vehicles.

A 2012 article in the "British Medical Journal" cited a study concluding that people who drive within three hours of using cannabis are dangerous behind the wheel.

The research concluded that while high on marijuana such individuals are twice as likely to cause an accident than drivers who had refrained from using any drugs.

Various other reports also have concluded that people who drive after using cannabis have an increased chance of accidents involving injuries.

According to a scientific report issued in 2013, at least 15 types of the drugs that were studied each caused a "modest" increase in the odds of an injurious or fatal accident.

But the report said that "compared to the huge increase in accident risk associated with alcohol, as well as the high accident rate among young drivers, the increases in risk associated with the use of (cannabis) drugs are surprisingly small."

As if to back up those findings, a 2015 report by the National Highway Traffic Safety Administration indicated that people using marijuana tend to have a much lower risk of vehicular accidents.

On February 15, 2015, the "Washington Post" said that the federal report concluded: "Drivers who tested positive for marijuana were no more likely to crash than (those individuals) who had not used any drugs or alcohol prior to driving."

18
Marijuana: The Unique, Natural & Safe Drug

Contrary to a worldwide misconception, marijuana hails as among the safest natural drugs--particularly when used by adults in moderate, non-excessive amounts.

Marijuana has a whopping 483 known compounds, according to "Cannabis and Cannabinoids: Pharmacology, Toxicology and Therapeutic Potential."

Written by Ethan B. Russo and published in 2002 by Routledge, the book lists 483 compounds in marijuana; a whopping 85 are within the cannabinoid class of diverse chemical compounds.

Inside the brain, these chemical compounds interact in perfect synchronization with what scientists call "cannabinoid receptors" in the body's natural cells.

To the delight of most marijuana users, these bodily receptors and microscopic plant structures interact in a "perfect, natural fit"--almost as if Mother Nature intended people to use and benefit from the drug.

Enlightened Discoveries Emerged

Scientists had an incorrect theory of marijuana's interaction with the body, until the 1980s. To that point researchers had incorrectly assumed that a non-specific interaction with cell membranes generated the behavioral and physiological effects of marijuana.

Yet according to a 2006 article in "Pharmacological Reviews," researchers in the 1980s determined that cannabis interacts with specific membrane-bound receptors.

These specific receptors are commonly found in animals including birds, reptiles, fish and mammals. These biological characteristics remain universal among animals.

After intense study, scientists were able to identify two unique types of cannabinoid receptors within these natural biological characteristics:

CB1 receptors: Located primarily within the peripheral and central nervous system, these receptors interact with cannabinoids including the psychoactive THC.

CB2 receptors: Even more than CB1 receptors, these play an essential role at enabling the body to interact with THC and the body's immune system.

To most people these details might seem highly complex and scientific. Yet each factor plays an important role in the medicinal effects that marijuana generates.

These attributes have emerged as so essential in the effectiveness of cannabis that some scientists believe that they'll eventually discover even more vital receptors.

Important Cancer-Fighting Attributes

While the attributes of CB1 receptors remain vital, the immune-enhancing attributes of CB2 receptors play a remarkable role in battling invaders such as cancer.

Scientists have found and carefully categorized CB2 receptors within various areas of the body's complex and inter-working overall immune system.

The thymus gland, spleen and tonsils are among these immune-boosting features, individually and collectively critical in producing cytokine that fight invading cells.

Necessary to achieve or to maintain overall good health, cytokines that "perfectly and ideally interact" with cannabinoid receptors include:

Monocytes: The largest of all leukocytes, these play multiple roles in immune function--particularly fighting inflammation and infection at specific bodily locations. The spleen stores half of them, ready for instant release into the body when needed.

Macrophages: These protective white blood cells strive to engulf and ingest cellular debris and other foreign substances including cancer cells. Microphages assist in the body's innate immunity, the so-called "first-line of defense." In addition, microphages ignite adaptive immunity, highly specialized cells ideal for fighting specific invaders.

B-Cells: These are different from other invader-fighting cells due to a protein surrounding the outer surface called a "B Cell Receptor." This unique attribute gives B-Cells the ability to bind to specific antigen, including certain otherwise harmful cells or substances such as cancer that sometimes start within the body.

T-Cells: Sometimes called "T lymphocytes," these mature in the thymus and sometimes the tonsils. Each of the various subsets of the T-Cell category, including "natural killer cells," has a unique function. Each actively seeks to find and destroy bodily invaders that if left unchecked would wreck or destroy good health, even causing death.

Cannabinoids Enhance Effectiveness

A vast array of scientific studies have independently concluded that cannabinoid receptors effectively bind with effective immune-boosting cells.

Reports and scientific papers detail these findings, printed in publications like the "Journal of Immunology" and the "European Journal of Biochemistry."

Besides immune function, the CB2 receptors play a critical role within the gastrointestinal system, where therapeutic targets include inflammatory bowel diseases.

CB2 receptors also have an impact within the brain, although not nearly as significant as CB1 receptors within that region.

The CB2 receptors within the brain primarily involve microglia cells, which comprise from 10 percent to 15 percent of that organ's mass. This factor emerges as important because the microglia--which also inhabit the spinal cord--serve as the central nervous system's primary and initial weaponry in active immune defense.

Scientists believe that partly due to these factors when interacting within the immune system the CB2 receptors likely assist in treatments for pain and inflammation.

Address Neurodegenerative Disorders

According to a 2003 article in the "Journal of Neuroscience," CB2 receptors likely have a significant role in treating neurodegenerative disorders like Alzheimer's disease.

A 2004 article in "Neurology" lists a suspected cause of Alzheimer's disease as the generation of beta-amyloid proteins or "senile plaques" that disrupt neural functioning.

This likely can be counteracted by using cannabis as an "agonist" or chemical to bind CB2 receptors, inducing macrophages to remove harmful beta-amyloid proteins.

As with many types of therapeutic applications involving marijuana, much more study needs to be done the drug's potential effectiveness within this area.

Hopefully scientists will launch far more extensive research within this area, as increasing numbers of states and local communities legalize recreational marijuana.

Another Unique Role

While CB2 receptors primarily involve the immune system's generators throughout the body, most human CB1 receptors are located within the brain.

Many of these cells are within the limbic system that regulates emotion, motivation, behavior, long-term memory and the critical ability to smell. Doctors believe that most of an individual's emotional life is located within the limbic system.

This emerges as extremely important from the perspective of marijuana users, particularly those wanting terrific, enjoyable highs made possible by THC.

Amazingly, the "medulla oblongata," the portion of the brain that regulates respiratory and cardiovascular functions, has no CB1 receptors.

Thus, some scientists believe the moderate or even heavy use of marijuana has little or no detrimental impact on blood pressure, breathing and heart rate. This unique attribute reportedly prevents marijuana from causing "death by overdose," a notorious outcome frequently caused by such dangerous drugs as heroin and barbiturates.

Extensive Diversity Exists

Remember that as previously mentioned, each marijuana plant has a whopping 85 different types of cannabinoids.

In what many people would consider a "blessing from Mother Nature," each of these specific structures generates a unique biological interaction within the human body.

Research scientists continue studying them all, particularly THC and:

Cannabidiol: Lacking the extensive psychoactive attributes of THC, this comprises a whopping 40 percent of the substance extracted from a cannabis plant. Many doctors insist that cannabidiol, sometimes called "CBD," possesses a far wider range of medical applications than THC. Within the United States, pharmaceutical companies distribute concentrated forms of CBD as an "orphan drug," the designation for chemical products produced to address extremely rare medical conditions. Under the brand name Epidiolex, concentrated CBD serves as an orally administered liquid for treating the previously mentioned Dravet syndrome--a severe myoclonic epilepsy, triggered by elevated fevers among infants. On the positive side, research indicates that high concentrations of CBD fail to generate short-term memory problems like those induced by THC. In fact, some studies indicate that CBD might serve as nature's way of counteracting the effects of THC on "psychosis," a general term referring to an "abnormal condition of the mind." For this very reason--the ability to counteract psychosis--CBD is a potentially effective treatment for people suffering from schizophrenia. Additionally, according to a 2011 article in "Neuropsychopharmacology," CBD reduces anxiety among people suffering from "social anxiety disorder." In addition, several other scientific and medical publications have published articles indicating that CBD serves as as an effective natural anti-depressant. Yet according to a 2012 article in the "Los Angeles Times," the typical percentages of CBD in cannabis plants began to decrease nationwide due to selective-breeding by growers. Eager to meet the demands from consumers motivated to get "high," these entrepreneurs worked to decrease CBD content while boosting THC levels. However, the increased demand for the health-enhancing attributes of CBD has motivated some marijuana harvesters to boost those levels in their crops--sometimes intended primarily for medicinal purposes. Partly as a result of these subtle--yet important--differences in cannabis strains, some drug companies have filed for patents on unique marijuana species that they have developed--strains not found in nature. Since 2005 under the brand name Sativex in Canada, physicians have prescribed an oral product with a 1:1 ratio of CBD and THC for alleviating pain from multiple sclerosis.

Cannabinol: Unlike the previously mentioned subset, cannabinol is found in only trace amounts in the two species--Cannabis sativa and Cannabis indica. Although relatively weak when interacting with CB1 receptors, cannabinol interacts much more readily with the important CB2 receptors that play a crucial role in the overall immune system. Cannabinol is "somewhat selective" in the CB2 receptors that it effectively interacts with. As a result, scientists are interested in studying cannabinol as a possible immunosuppressant, actually reducing the effectiveness or "efficacy" of the immune system. Such drugs are used to counteract unique or challenging medical or biological situations, such as preventing the body from rejecting a transplanted organ. Scientists also are interested in the possibility of using cannabinol in addressing auto-immune ailments such as Crohn's disease-- an inflammatory bowel condition. Amazingly, although derived from marijuana plants, this substance sometimes called "CBN," is legal to possess, buy and sell on the United States' federal level; cannabinol is not listed on the federal "schedule" of illegal drugs. However, readers should be forewarned that cannabinol might be considered as having a chemical analog or structure similar to the THC psychoactive byproduct of marijuana. This characteristic would make cannabinol illegal under the Federal Analogue Act; passed in 1986 as part of the Controlled Substances Act, this regulates substances deemed "substantially similar" to chemicals listed as illegal in Schedule I and Schedule II of the regulations.

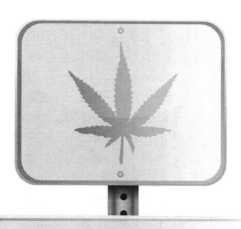

DO NOT MIX
WITH OTHER DRUGS

19
Warning: The Extreme Dangers of "Poly Drug Use"

Health professionals and even some long-time advocates of psychoactive cannabis strongly warn against mixing or using marijuana with other drugs--particularly those in the psychoactive category.

The strong sense of urgency focuses on the fact that scientists admittedly lack sufficient knowledge about the dangers of mixing marijuana with other drugs.

This seems understandable, at least from the viewpoint of many people, largely due to the fact that--unlike marijuana--some psychoactive drugs are highly addictive.

Besides so-called "natural" substances like heroin or opium, this warning holds true for many brands of unnatural drugs such as painkillers produced by Big Pharma.

"Know what you're taking," marijuana users are sometimes told. "Never risk the possibility that someone has surreptitiously added other drugs to the cannabis that you buy. Always ask your seller, 'Is this pure weed? Is something else in here?'"

Just as essential, at least from the standpoint of health professionals, marijuana users also have a right to know if "chemicals other than natural fertilizers" were used to nourish and help grow cannabis plants. For the most part, scientists reportedly lack sufficient data on the possible health dangers of smoking or eating such chemicals.

Assured Safety Benefits
People who advocate legalized marijuana argue that removing

prohibitions against the drug promotes safety. This way, they say, "consumers will know what they're actually purchasing, in a licensed and government-monitored facility."

Any dispensary that sells tainted cannabis would risk having its license revoked by authorities, while consumers buying in the "underground market" lack such protections.

Authorities have no data on the percentage of marijuana that has been infused with other illicit drugs sold in the underground market. Officials also lack reliable data regarding the number of such overdoses.

Mindful of these extreme dangers, people who want to buy pure marijuana should ask themselves questions like, "Do I know and trust this seller well enough?" and "What other kinds of drugs, if any, does this person sell?"

A seller who admits to providing other types of illegal drugs might have the potential for clandestine mixing. An additional possible danger might arise, if it's true what some law enforcement authorities insist about marijuana; they call cannabis "a doorway drug."

Briefly mentioned earlier, this term signifies the supposed danger that people who initially use and like marijuana are far more likely to eventually start abusing and becoming addicted to other illicit drugs deemed far more dangerous than psychoactive cannabis. Marijuana advocates insist such claims are "mere poppycock," while as previously mentioned some politicians and law enforcement officials argue that as a "doorway drug," this famous substance poses extreme danger.

The Intentional Mixing of Drugs

Despite the many strong warnings against doing so, an undetermined number of psychoactive cannabis users intentionally mix marijuana with other drugs including alcohol. This practice is called "poly drug use," sometimes with the first two words joined as "polydrug."

Although alcohol is sometimes involved, the term polydrug technically involves a mixture of two or more psychoactive drugs. These chemical substances change brain function, invariably altering consciousness, mood and perceptions.

A wide variety of drugs listed as psychoactive provide what mainstream doctors consider legitimate purposes, everything from painkillers to treating convulsions, neuro-psychiatric disorders and many other adverse health conditions.

Scientists lack any significant data and conclusions on the body's likely reactions to these many potential mixtures. In almost every instance, however, scientists seem to agree that extreme dangers emerge from "poly drug" use. This is particularly true when haphazardly mixing a wide variety of psychoactive drugs for recreational purposes.

Specifics on mixing the THC psychoactive ingredient with alcohol also seem difficult to pinpoint, largely due to the apparent lack of reliable studies.

The psychoactive category of narcotics includes extremely dangerous and highly addictive psychedelic drugs including LSD, psilocybin mushrooms, and mescaline. Drugs in crystalline form include cocaine and methamphetamine.

Although widely discussed as a topic of established scientific literature for instances where standard drugs are involved, marijuana is rarely discussed in-depth and often never mentioned in such scientific papers.

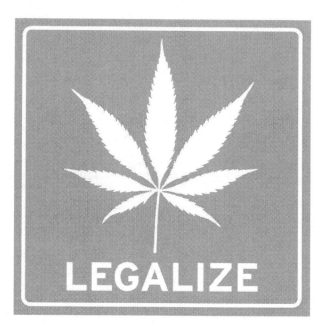

20

Legalized Marijuana: The Fastest-Growing Industry

The growth, distribution and sale of legalized marijuana for recreational and medicinal purposes has rapidly grown into the fastest-growing industry in the United States, according to a 2015 report by the Arc View Group, which provides financial news and data on legal cannabis markets.

Streams of companies dedicated to generating profit from legalized marijuana businesses started trading in the securities industry, with steadily increasing frequency during the second decade of the 21st Century.

The onslaught of surging consumer demand for marijuana products also sharply increased interest in getting jobs in the industry. To help job seekers, several companies launched apps that enable people to find cannabis-related employment.

The growing stream of apps include software available via WeedHire.com, Cannajobs.com, and 420Careers.com.

"Marijuana is no different than other industries, and its not just about the plant," WeedHire founder David Bernstein told Yahoo Business News in April 2015. "There's a need for people to work in accounting, finance, legal, HR" and other positions.

Cannabis Fuels the Economy

Whether or not anti-marijuana advocates like to admit this, legalization of the drug has rapidly boosted numerous regional economies in the United States--particularly in Colorado, among the first states to permit recreational use of the drug.

By late 2014, just a few years after marijuana became legal

when grown for and sold at government-authorized dispensaries in Colorado, a whopping 15,992 people had obtained licenses to work in such facilities in that state.

As that total continued to grow, tens of thousands of similar jobs were either being filled or scheduled for openings in other states in the process of legalizing recreational cannabis.

Once these proverbial floodgates opened, citizens of numerous other states aggressively advocated similar legalization in their communities. Seemingly no one wanted to get left behind as a proverbial freight train representing the rapid growth of the marijuana industry continued accelerating nationwide.

Salaries for many cannabis industry jobs soared much higher than the maximum national poverty rate of less than about $12,000 to $20,000 per individual. Licensed marijuana industry salaries surpassed $100,000 for positions requiring specialized degrees, such as epidemiologists.

Specialized Companies Flourished

Energized by a sharp increase in demand for legal marijuana, the stock prices of many cannabis-related companies sharply increased through first quarter of 2015.

At least four such companies benefited in March of that year by "making headway in the development of their brands within this growing market," according to a story posted by the AccessWire News Service.

"If you were in the market last year, you'll vividly remember the drop in share prices that many marijuana stocks had due to stringent regulation and even stock halts," the 2015 article said. "What that has created is a more savvy and informed public and on the same token, a generally more transparent group of publicly traded marijuana companies working hard to play by the rules."

According to AccessWire, these companies included:

Blue Line Protection Group: Traded under the symbol BLPG on the Over the Counter market, Blue Line Protection Group is described in its press releases as "a leader in providing regulatory compliance, security consultation and protection services to high-value asset industries." In April 2015, the company announced that it ensures safe, lawful cannabis operations in downtown Denver's retail district. Details: BlueLineProtectionGroup.com

Totally Hemp Crazy Inc: Traded with the symbol THCZ on the Over the Counter market, this firm's Website says that the company produces and sells hemp energy drinks, hemp lemonade, and hemp iced tea. Details: TotallyHempCrazy.com

PharmaCyte Biotech Inc: Traded with the symbol PMBC on the Over the Counter market, this company is described in its press releases as a clinical stage biotechnology company focused on developing and preparing treatments for cancer and diabetes. According to this company's Website, its goal is to combine the Cell-in-a-Box(r) cellulose-based live cell encapsulation technology with constituents of cannabis to develop "unique treatments for difficult-to-treat deadly forms of cancer." Details: PharmaCyteBiotech.com.

Investors Have Options

As with all stocks, any investment involves risk when involving companies that specialize in the marijuana industry. Largely for this reason, no particular companies are recommended here for investment purposes. Potential investors in marijuana companies need to conduct their own research, or seek the help of a licensed securities expert or financial adviser.

The brief list of companies already mentioned here are only a handful of the many publicly traded marijuana-related firms.

Additionally, lots of these companies are listed as "penny stocks," technically any security that trades at less than $5 per share. Some financial analysts consider penny stocks as highly speculative.

All along, just like mainstream stocks, the shares of marijuana companies as an overall group are sometimes unpopular or popular for intermittent periods.

During the spring of 2015, Yahoo's cannabis industry analysis said, "it would seem, for now, that the sentiment surrounding marijuana stocks has begun to turn positive and this can also be echoed in many segments of the marketing including the biotech segment."

Even so, by the time some potential investors first learn of supposedly "hot" cannabis stocks, market sentiments might have soured. Also, a percentage of start-up companies eventually fold in almost every industry, while a limited number of firms move forward in generating steady and solid financial growth.

21
Marijuana and Hemp: History Throughout Society

Marijuana and hemp products have had a complex and diverse history throughout societies worldwide since modern civilizations began 10,000 years ago.

The numerous strains of cannabis and methods for using them have become so diverse worldwide that literally hundreds of terms have been coined to describe users, varieties and strategies.

The hundreds of distinct and unique strains have ranged from the Acapulco gold and African bush strains to Maui-Wauie and Jamaican gold.

One of the most popular and frequently used slang terms, "weed," refers to the fact that marijuana grows wildly on a rapid and unchecked basis throughout nature.

Luckily from the perspective of cannabis users, its unique, natural and wild-growing qualities have made the plant difficult if not impossible for authorities to fully destroy worldwide.

The many dozens of slang terms that refer to marijuana in general range from Mary Jane and Mary to Meg, Mother and Giggle Smoke. The Jamaican word for cannabis, "Ganja," has become so widespread that many users in the United States prefer the term.

Many People Ignored the Laws

Motivated by the euphoric high and a sense of peace provided by marijuana, people in many cultures have ignored laws prohibiting the use and sale of the drug.

Frequent marijuana users sometimes get saddled with the

label "pothead," a weed user's equivalent of an alcoholic. Most potheads and alcoholics are--or have been--frequent and non-stop users of their drug of choice.

From a medical standpoint, marijuana is far less harmful to the human body than alcohol. Remember, particularly when used under the proper medical guidance of a licensed physician, cannabis can emerge as highly beneficial to the body and mind.

By contrast, excessive alcohol consumption sometimes leads to destruction of the essential liver organ, generating cirrhosis that often results in death.

Tragically adding to these dangers, every day worldwide people die of alcohol overdoses when excessively consumed in large amounts during short or extended periods. Excessive levels of alcohol in the blood stream shut down or hamper brain function, leading to organ failure.

Also, remember the aforementioned fact that advocates of cannabis sometimes proclaim, particularly during public forums on the issue, that "No one in human history has ever died of a marijuana overdose."

Although such statements might seem ludicrous to novices or people misinformed about the issue, marijuana--even when consumed in high quantities--has a far lower propensity than alcohol to shut down vital organ function.

Early Humans Lacked Such Prohibitions

Humans have found and used marijuana as recently as the end of the last Ice Age, shortly after glaciers melted and many climates warmed worldwide.

Archaeologists and historians claim that they can pinpoint the start of marijuana's worldwide use to the earliest Chinese and Viking cultures.

According to numerous published reports, the earliest use of cannabis on a widespread scale can be tracked to what is now the Chinese region of East Asia.

Even way back then, before the advent of today's most popular religions, the earliest cultures that used marijuana did so at least partly for spiritual reasons.

Yet just as important from the standpoint of today's pro-cannabis advocates, the earliest users of weed also did so for medicinal purposes. The obvious health benefits became apparent almost right away among many of these ancient cultures..

Early Societies Lacked Restrictions

Numerous news reports in late 2014 quoted Barney Wharf, a professor of geography at the University of Kansas, as saying that the Vikings and medieval Germans used cannabis to relieve childbirth and toothache pain.

"The idea that this is an evil drug is a very recent construction," Wharf was quoted as saying. From his perspective the criminalization of cannabis is a "historical anomaly."

Adding to the overall international confusion on this issue, gradually over time many people became confused regarding the four distinctive subspecies of cannabis:

Cannabis sativa: This is the plant that generates a euphoric psychoactive high, famous and even notorious in some societies.

Cannabis sativa L: Commonly known as hemp when 100-percent pure and non-flowering, this lacks psychoactive attributes--yet useful in manufacturing various products like fuel cloth and oil. The letter "L" was added to this subspecies, honoring botanist Carl Linnaeus.

Cannabis indica: Jean-Baptiste Lamarck, a French naturalist, discovered this subspecies, which has a distinctive, unique psychoactive quality. In its rare, pure form this is classified as "hemp," but only when having THC levels that are significantly lower than 1 percent.

Cannabis ruderalis: Less common than the other subspecies, this also has a psychoactive effect; Russian botanist D.E. Janischevisky named this in 1924.

Marijuana Became Early Crop

Today's anti-cannabis groups might dislike reading this, but anthropologists claim that thousands of years ago marijuana became one of the first crops ever grown.

Marijuana farming spread as people in a steadily growing numbers of cultures experienced the mental and bodily benefits derived from this miraculous natural substance.

According to news interviews that Wharf granted, and his scientific papers, people first discovered cannabis in central Asia thousands of years before Christ.

Perhaps as long as 12,000 years ago people within the regions of southern Siberia and Mongolia discovered to their delight that cannabis generates a mild or even intense euphoria.

Motivated to get high as much as possible, early hunters and gatherers noticed to their delight that marijuana grew heartily at nutrient-rich dump sites. The earliest modern-era humans used these places to discard dead plants and carcasses.

Gradually over time people worked to modify and strengthen the psychoactive potency of the various subspecies of marijuana.

Medicinal Qualities Became High Priority

Within ancient China the many medicinal qualities of marijuana became a priority 6,000 years ago--about 4,000 years before Christ.

Shortly after accepting cannabis for its health-enhancing attributes, the early Chinese began leaving marijuana at burial grounds and within the tombs of nobles.

Marijuana became so accepted deep within early Chinese culture that mourners placed large quantities of mummified marijuana within some tombs.

By this point many people throughout that ancient culture considered cannabis as a phenomenal herb, vital as a powerful and life-saving anesthetic during surgery.

This socially acceptable practice continued 2,000 years before

Christ, to the point when Aryans started invading China. The invaders then took some marijuana to India, while speaking an Indo-European language considered archaic today.

Cannabis Quickly Became Popular Throughout India

Marijuana apparently surged in popularity throughout India shortly after its introduction into that culture about 4,000 years ago.

Authorities refrained from imposing restrictions on cannabis throughout that region and then during subsequent transformations into numerous European cultures.

"Health experts" within India's ancient culture quickly categorized cannabis as one of the Kingdoms of Herbs. Heralded for their substantial abilities at relieving stress, the herbs included lemon balm, kava, valerian root, passionflower, and St. John's Wort.

From India, cannabis moved to the Middle East, apparently used there by Eurasian nomads sometimes called "Scythians." From about 2,000 years to 1,400 years before Christ, this Indo-European group transported cannabis to the Ukraine and Russia.

As positive word-of-mouth spread about cannabis, the drug then spread from Eastern Europe into early Germanic tribes who eagerly took the plant back home to Germany.

Nearly 1,000 years later, about 500 years after Christ, the Anglo-Saxons took cannabis into the future Britain when invading those lands and early cultures.

Marijuana Spread on a Worldwide Scale

Cannabis was readily accepted and used from that point forward, thanks to its psychoactive qualities, coupled with an ability to address medical problems,

Sociologists and anthropologists say that from about 1,200 years to 1,800 years after Christ, cannabis spread from Europe, southward along Eastern Africa.

By 1400 a.d., marijuana had spread to the extreme southern tip of Africa, in a region now known as Johannesburg.

To that point virtually every culture where cannabis emerged quickly accepted and embraced the plant, which earned a well-deserved reputation as natural and harmless.

Amazingly, however, Wharf reported that cannabis never spread directly from Europe into the New World. The specific reason apparently remains unclear.

Long after Christopher Columbus initially landed in the Americas in 1492, in the 1600s through the early 1800s marijuana was shipped west from South Africa.

These initial shipments or "migrations" of cannabis went north along Africa's western edge, before going to Brazil and the Caribbean.

Cannabis Moved Northward

From Peru, marijuana gradually spread north through Central America, where the weed naturally grew and spread in abundance throughout tropical environments.

According to Wharf, cannabis finally entered the United States when carried by Mexicans nearly 50 years after the American Civil War.

Wharf believes that migrants fleeing the Mexican Revolution carried cannabis to the American Southwest regions of Arizona and New Mexico in 1910 and 1911.

Strangely, this critical juncture in marijuana's worldwide evolution marked the first time that any nation imposed widespread anti-cannabis laws.

"Many early prejudices against marijuana were thinly veiled racist fears of its smokers, often promulgated by reactionary newspapers," Wharf wrote.

These inflammatory news stories helped fan the initial flames of American ignorance regarding the many natural health-enhancing benefits of cannabis.

Instead of recognizing the many positive, health-enhancing attributes of marijuana, the ill-informed white journalists printed streams of explosive stories about the what they called "loco" Mexicans.

These highly inflammatory articles claimed that marijuana-smoking Mexicans who moved into the American Southwest went on wild murder sprees and sexually assaulted women and children.

The mainstream American public considered marijuana "strange" at the time. According to the racist stories spread rampantly by the news media during the first few decades of the 1900s, the plant supposedly transformed Mexicans into wickedly violent and sub-human animals. These shockingly untrue, racist articles spread nationwide, fanning the political calls to criminalize marijuana.

Anti-Marijuana LAWS

22
America's Harsh
Anti-Marijuana Laws

In an odd and seemingly bizarre twist, the earliest governments of the future United States began allowing non-psychoactive hemp in the early 1600s.

Nearly 300 years before Mexicans first brought psychoactive cannabis into the American Southwest, the Virginia Legislature required all farmers to grow hemp.

Deemed useful at creating various products and valuable for trade purposes, authorities allowed exchanges of hemp in Maryland, Virginia and Pennsylvania.

Hemp production and trade flourished throughout that region until shortly after the Civil War, when various products and imports overtook the plant in popularity.

Meantime, according to the Public Broadcasting System, psychoactive marijuana became an ingredient in medicinal products sold in U.S. pharmacies.

Yet for the most part the general public throughout those early years in U.S. history remained relatively unaware of the existence of psychoactive marijuana.

Even so, through the 19th Century smoking "hash" containing psychoactive attributes of cannabis became a fad in France and to a limited degree in the U.S.

Authorities Initially Accepted Marijuana

In 1906, just five or six years before racist reports about Mexicans harmed the drug's nationwide reputation, Congress passed the Pure Food and Drug Act.

By passing this law, the nation's top elected leaders readily welcomed and accepted psychoactive marijuana into the American culture during the administration of Republican President Theodore "Teddy" Roosevelt.

The only requirement stipulated that over-the-counter remedies containing this natural substance featured labels that told consumers of the cannabinoid content.

Although on a relatively low behind-the-scenes scale, this overall acceptance of psychoactive cannabis gradually changed when the Mexican issue erupted nationwide.

Within the mindset of "mainstream white Americans" at the time, relatively all Spanish-speaking immigrants from Mexico were associated with marijuana.

U.S. citizens opposed to drugs, particularly religious zealots, began referring to the issue and to the Mexicans as the "Marijuana Menace."

Fear of Mexican Immigrants

The unfounded and racist fears of Mexican immigrants intensified and spread throughout the mainstream U.S. culture in the 1910s through the Roaring '20s.

By the advent of the 1930s as the Great Depression walloped the economy, the level of racist attitudes against Mexican-Americans reached a fever pitch.

Adding to these problems multi-fold, bogus and irresponsible research wrongly concluded that marijuana sparks socially deviant behaviors including violent crime.

As if these deceptions were not enough, authorities embraced the irresponsible conclusion that marijuana use involved "racially inferior" underclass communities.

Primarily as a result, by 1931 at least 29 states had outlawed marijuana, two years before the repeal of the nation's 13-year Prohibition that had criminalized and prohibited alcohol.

At that point the initial groundwork had been set, putting the nation on a misguided pathway leading to an eventual federal ban on marijuana.

Ludicrous Laws Intensified

The ludicrous, inane and cruel laws imposed by individual states intensified. Some offenders were jailed up to one decade just for smoking a single joint.

Sadly, such criminal convictions occurred even though marijuana is a relatively harmless substance, except when used irresponsibly such as before driving.

Rather than imposing sensible regulations that punish people who drive while high on psychoactive cannabis or people who sell the drug to children, lawmakers in many states classified marijuana use,sales, possession and production as a felony.

Contrary to the misguided beliefs of politicians at the time, using marijuana rarely causes people to become violent criminals or sexual deviants.

Instead, marijuana generates a mild or intense sense of euphoria. Often referred to as a "high," this condition involves a sense of peace and tranquility--relieving mental tension.

People rarely exhibit anger or violence when high on marijuana. By contrast, alcohol often generates the opposite behaviors in some people, such as violent fistfights.

Rampant Alcohol Use Resumed

Just as many people had feared, alcohol consumption rapidly intensified nationwide soon after the 1933 passage of the 21st Amendment made booze legal again.

Particularly since then, a maze of disturbing data has shown that alcohol has had a dangerous, detrimental impact on U.S. society--including health, causing death and destroying families.

According to a variety of studies and medical reports, cannabis has a far less disastrous impact than alcohol on life expectancies and health.

Even today, any negative impacts generated by marijuana receive far less media coverage than the rampant problems caused by alcohol.

The societal destruction generated by booze has been well documented, steadily worsening on a grand scale during the more than 80 years since Prohibition ended.

Traffic deaths: Hundreds of thousands of Americans have died in alcohol-related vehicle accidents. During 2013, a whopping 10,076 people including children and entire families died in such accidents in the United States, according to the non-profit Mothers Against Drunk Driving organization.

Alcohol deaths: Each year from the beginning of 2006 through 2010 an average of 88,000 people died from alcohol; 440,000 died from this cause during the five-year period, according to the U.S. Centers for Disease Control (CDC). The specific underlying causes included overdoses and livers damaged by excessive, long-term alcohol consumption.

Death rate: A disturbing one out of every 10 people who die yearly between ages 20 and 64 perish as a result of alcohol consumption.

Economic destruction: Alcohol related deaths rob the U.S. economy of tens of billions of dollars from the overall economy. The CDC estimates that the 88,000 people who die yearly would have lived a combined 2.5 million additional years; over the five-year span a total 12.5 million years of life were lost.

Everyone suffers: Almost as if mimicking the Grim Reaper, the destruction caused by alcohol fails to play favorites. Alcoholism and alcohol-related deaths ravage all of society, every race and religion--from the poor to the ultra-rich, the very young to the extremely old.

Helpful Organization: Founded in 1935 two years after Prohibition ended, the mutual-aid fellowship Alcoholics Anonymous assists alcoholics in their ongoing battle to avoid booze. Commonly known as "AA," the fellowship announced in 2001 that worldwide membership had reached more than 2 million. The work each alcoholic must endure to remain sober involves a continual, uninterrupted lifetime commitment. Yet sadly, only 26 percent of people who first go to an AA meeting are still attending the organization's sessions one year later, according to the "Cochran Database of Systematic Reviews."

Differing Addiction Levels

When compared on a scientific basis, alcohol and psychoactive cannabis have vastly different addiction levels.

A September 2014 issue of "The Atlantic" mentioned studies showing that the lifetime risk of addiction to marijuana is lower than most drugs.

On an overall basis, nicotine is by far the most addictive, followed respectively by heroin, cocaine and alcohol. Marijuana comes in last place in this category, by far the least addictive.

However, any claim that the drug should be considered 100-percent safe in all instances is dubious at best. Ordinarily harmless substances such as water can generate fatal overdoses when consumed in massive amounts over short periods of time.

With equal importance, if these studies are accurate, 15 percent of alcohol users become addicted to that substance. Studies reveal that by comparison just 9 percent of marijuana users generate an addiction to psychoactive cannabis.

Intense Debate Continues

The debate on whether pot or booze is safer likely will continue for many more generations, although alcohol hails as far more dangerous and deadly in every regard.

Another intrinsic factor involves the availability of drugs. At least one official at the National Institute on Drug Abuse has said that nicotine likely has gained a reputation as the "most addictive" due to the widespread availability of tobacco products.

By contrast, for many consumers heroin, cocaine and marijuana are much more challenging than tobacco products to locate and acquire. This low-accessibility factor, in turn, might result in conclusions that indicate those drugs have much higher probabilities of causing addiction--when compared to alcohol and marijuana.

Yet some researchers believe that as more states legalize recreational and medicinal marijuana, the availability of cannabis will sharply increase in those jurisdictions.

Over time, they say, this changing factor in turn could very well result in an increase in the perceived percentage of people who become addicted to marijuana.

Overall Safety Issue

Besides addiction rates, the overall controversy likely will continue concerning whether marijuana is generally safe when regularly consumed at moderate levels.

Remember that as previously indicated marijuana use should never be considered completely risk-free in all instances.

According to federal government statistics as reported by the "Washington Post," marijuana generated a half million Emergency Room visits in 2011.

However, according to the National Institutes of Health, marijuana generated far fewer ER visits than heroin, cocaine, meth and alcohol.

In fact, these statistics show that extremely dangerous prescription drugs made by pharmaceutical companies and prescribed by doctors are far more dangerous than marijuana.

Federal data also indicate that out of every 1,000 marijuana users, only 27 visited Emergency Rooms. But from among every 1,000 pharmaceutical-drug users, 111 went to the ER, more than four times the rate of hospitalized marijuana users.

As expected, the overall rate of ER visits becomes far more disturbing when heroin becomes involved. Of every 1,000 users of that substance, a whopping 940 eventually end up in the Emergency Room, according the National Institutes of Health.

Other ER-visit rates per 1,000 users of each substance during 2011 were: cocaine, 325; methamphetamine, 292; and alcohol, 35.

Ultimately, the "Washington Post" said, "Alcohol is about 30 percent more likely to send you to the ER than marijuana. These are the federal government's own numbers, and they show that marijuana is considerably less harmful to users than alcohol."

Alcohol Problems Intensify

U.S. citizens abuse alcohol at a far greater level than any other drug.

A mind-boggling 17.6 million people, or about 1 out of every 12 adults in the United States suffer from alcohol abuse or dependence, according to the National Institute of Alcohol Abuse and Alcoholism.

Additional disturbing data were generated by the National Institute on Drug Abuse. That federal agency concludes that only 9 percent of marijuana users become addicted to psychoactive cannabis, while 20 percent of cocaine users became addicted.

"There is clear evidence that in some people marijuana can lead to withdrawal symptoms, including insomnia, anxiety and nausea," Doctor Sanjay Gupta, chief medical correspondent at CNN, wrote in his previously mentioned article, "Why I Changed my Mind on Weed."

To his credit, Gupta wrote that even considering the occasional marijuana withdrawal issues, "it is hard to make a case that it has a high potential for abuse. The physical symptoms of marijuana addiction are nothing like those of the other drugs that I have mentioned."

Public Awareness Sharply Increased Demand

Voters in at least five states were scheduled to decide during the 2016 general elections whether to legalize recreational marijuana in those jurisdictions.

Many analysts predicted victory for the pro-cannabis crowd.

Florida voters were among those who signed enough petitions to authorize a 2016 ballot to legalize medicinal marijuana.

Upon seeing a sharp increase in public sentiment to allow such prescriptions, Republicans in Florida's legislature did a quick about-face on the issue in early 2015.

After opposing such efforts through 2014, the Republican lawmakers quickly crafted legislation to broaden Florida's medical marijuana laws.

According to ABC News, political analysts concluded that GOP legislators were merely bowing to a growing tide of intense public sentiment favoring marijuana.

By early 2015, legislators in 23 states had already passed laws allowing medical cannabis; Florida would become the first Southern state with such regulations.

23
Warped Federal Perspective

The federal government refrained from relaxing its anti-marijuana stance, despite such solid and steadily increasing public sentiment favoring the drug.

The U.S. Drug Enforcement Administration lists this natural drug as a notorious Schedule I substance--along with hard-core drugs like LSD, heroin and ecstasy.

This warped bureaucratic perspective toward marijuana has robbed many people of the significant benefits provided by medicinal cannabis.

Equally disturbing, although proven as far more harmful and more addictive than psychoactive cannabis, alcohol is legal nationwide for everyone at least age 21. Some states have legalized alcohol for people as young as 18.

Considering these disturbing facts, many key questions arise that spark numerous intriguing and perplexing issues.

For instance, what would society be like today if in 1933 when Prohibition ended, U.S. authorities had instead legalized marijuana--while criminalizing alcohol?

Magical Hypothetical Situations

Imagine going into a typical U.S. grocery store today, to find absolutely no alcohol--but rather an entire aisle dedicated to the marijuana sales.

At least from the perspective of many of today's average consumers, such a scenario would provide far healthier options for society as a whole.

Of course, numerous studies in recent years have concluded

that moderate amounts of alcohol consumed daily have proven distinctive health benefits as well.

Yet while minimal daily amounts of alcohol might aid digestion and enhance heart function somewhat, absolutely no studies indicate that can "cure" cancer the way that weed oil apparently does.

Due to instances such as this, the U.S. government's draconic rules involving marijuana seem highly politicized--to the point of being overly extreme or even absurd.

The Feds Demonized Marijuana

Starting as soon as Prohibition ended, the federal government launched a full-scale legislative and propaganda campaign demonizing marijuana.

As previously mentioned, by that point in 1933 at least 29 states had outlawed marijuana, motivated by bogus, racist and misinformed perceptions of this natural plant.

Paving the way for this all-out war against the drug, in 1930 the U.S. government formed the Federal Bureau of Narcotics--a new law enforcement agency.

Soon afterward researchers closely allied to this federal bureaucracy concluded that marijuana use generated extremely violent behavior and rampant crime.

Today we know that such findings are ludicrous and irresponsible. By that point the damage that bureaucrats imposed on society was already well underway.

Yet rather than advocate federal legislation criminalizing marijuana nationwide, the Federal Bureau of Narcotics encouraged all states to strengthen anti-cannabis laws.

"Refer Madness" Propaganda Film

With the apparent blessing of U.S. federal officials, from 1936 to 1939 a church group financed production of the anti-marijuana propaganda film "Reefer Madness."

Produced by French filmmaker Louis J. Gasnier, the movie was crammed with misconceptions about marijuana--portrayed as resulting in addiction-fueled madness.

Ignorant about the issue and thereby misguided in their motivations, the church sponsoring the project originally intended to show the movie only to parents.

The film's morality tale centers on the tragic consequences suffered by a high school student that drug pushers convince to try marijuana. The young man becomes involved in a hit-and-run accident, manslaughter, rape, hallucinations and ultimately madness.

Originally entitled "Tell Your Children," rights to the film were eventually purchased by producer Dwain Esper, who promptly re-cut the footage.

Eager to profit from public hysteria and misinformation regarding the issue, Esper distributed the exploitation film from the late 1930s through the 1950s.

Many people who saw the movie during that era got fooled, convinced that the Devil created marijuana to condemn people to madness and hell.

In his 2005 book, "The History of Reefer Madness," Dan Studney describes how advocates of reforming marijuana laws "rediscovered" the film in the 1970s. That decade's critics panned the cult movie as among history's worst movies. Today's viewers consider the film hilarious; the movie can be seen for free online because the copyright has expired, thereby shifting the film into the public domain.

The Feds Remained Timid

By almost every account the federal government remained relatively timid on the marijuana issue from the 1930s through the 1960s.

Although the Federal Bureau of Narcotics continued encouraging states to enact anti-cannabis laws, the agency refrained from imposing those rules on the federal level.

Rather than flat-out ban marijuana nationwide, in 1937 Congress passed the wimpy Marijuana Tax Act, embracing nationwide propaganda against "the evil weed."

While refraining from a direct federal prohibition on marijuana, the new regulation effectively criminalized any widespread recreational use of the drug.

On the federal level, the law authorized the possession of marijuana, but only among people who paid an excise tax-- required when using the drug for medical or industrial purposes.

Officials Ignored Scientists

Swept up in a wave of public misconception on the issue, in 1944 near the end of World War II lawmakers ignored positive scientific findings regarding marijuana.

That year a research team at the New York Academy of Medicine concluded in its "La Guardia Report" that contrary to popular belief marijuana never induces violence.

Just as important, the researchers announced that cannabis never causes sex crimes, insanity, and addiction, nor does using it typically lead to the use of other drugs.

This decision by lawmakers to ignore positive scientific data regarding marijuana launched the "era of ignorance," bogus anti-cannabis propaganda information still embraced by many of today's ill-informed politicians.

With increasing intensity as the Cold War began in the late 1940s and early 1950s, the anti-marijuana bureaucracy reigned. Purely for political reasons rather than science-based facts, federal government officials continually adopted and enforced reckless and needless anti-marijuana laws through the last half of the 20th Century.

Hemp for Victory

As if parents dishing out mixed messages to their offspring, at the height of World War II the federal government launched a "Hemp for Victory" campaign.

Employing a hodgepodge of conflicting regulations, the U.S. Department of Agriculture gave hemp seeds to farmers and encouraged them to plant the crop.

This came about because through 1942, the first full calendar year of the war, officials realized that they lacked enough materials to make vital military supplies.

Like marijuana, hemp is part of the cannabis family of plants. Unlike marijuana, however, pure hemp lacks psychoactive attributes--commonly known as the THC ingredient that makes people high.

Through the early 1940s, authorities desperately needed enough hemp materials for the crucial production of parachutes, marine cordage and other vital military necessities.

The federal program emerged as successful when farmers nationwide harvested a whopping 375,000 acres of hemp. These materials contributed substantially to country's war effort.

Yet the paradoxical situation contributed to the overall widespread public misconception involving hemp and marijuana. The two species became intermingled in the minds of many Americans; streams of law-abiding citizens remained unaware that hemp generally lacks substantial amounts of psychoactive ingredients--never enough to "get high."

Thus, many average U.S. citizens mistakenly adopted an incorrect and ill-informed belief that "marijuana" rather than hemp had somehow played a significant and important role in winning the war.

Public Confusion Worsens

At least by some accounts, the overall public confusion and conflicting opinions regarding marijuana increased substantially during the 1950s and 1960s.

The first round of confusion occurred in 1956 when Congress passed the Boggs Act, imposing mandatory sentences for certain drug offenses including marijuana.

This new rule demonized use of the "evil weed," imposing minimum two to 10-year sentences for first-time marijuana possession--plus fines up to $20,000.

The tough new regulations soon entered a paradoxical situation the following decade, amid a burst in popularity for marijuana across much of the United States.

With steadily increasing intensity through the 1960s streams of young adults began using illicit drugs, particularly psychoactive cannabis.

That turbulent decade generated a wide divide between supporters of the Vietnam War and anti-war factions largely comprised of "dope-smoking, college-age hippies."

Through the late 1960s and early 1970s streams of older people, particularly conservatives, pushed for harsher anti-cannabis laws--perhaps at least in part to punish rebellious, dope-smoking young adults.

This period marked an increase in the popularity of psychologist Timothy Leary, who urged people to "turn on, tune in, drop out" by using drugs like LSD and marijuana.

Many Felt Shocked

The supposedly wild, hard-partying behaviors of Leary and people who adored his philosophies shocked many citizens who worried the country was losing its moral values.

During the late 1960s through the first several years of the 1970s, marijuana became linked with heroin and other dangerous drugs in the minds of many Americans.

Rock guitarist, singer and songwriter Jimi Hendrix died of a heroin overdose in September 1970 in London, England. Rock singer-songwriter Janis Joplin perished from a similar overdose

184

the next month in Hollywood. The following summer's death of The Doors band rocker Jim Morrison in Paris generated rumors of another apparent heroin overdose.

Tragic deaths such as these from a drug far more dangerous than marijuana indirectly increased the notoriety of cannabis. Many among the so-called "silent majority" of Americans over age 40 considered this drug as extremely dangerous like all narcotics, just as notorious as heroin.

Much to their credit, however, some congressmen agreed with scientific researchers who concluded that marijuana poses much less danger than most illegal drugs.

Largely as a result, in early 1970 the United States Congress briefly repealed the mandatory sentences for most drug-related federal offenses. According to the Public Broadcasting System, lawmakers believed that the mandatory and unduly harsh minimum sentences imposed since the 1950s had failed to eliminate the drug culture.

Restrictions Briefly Loosened

Rather than merely eliminate mandatory sentences for marijuana use and possession, Congress began categorizing cannabis separately from other narcotics.

These changes occurred as a result of the Comprehensive Drug Abuse, Prevention and Control Act of 1970, removing mandatory sentences for possessing small amounts.

Although refraining from an all-out legalization of marijuana, Congress made the wise and sensible decision to remove the overly harsh restrictions against this substance.

Encouraged by this change, the same year advocates of cannabis formed the non-profit National Association for the Reform of Marijuana Laws (NORML).

Still working diligently today on the domestic and international level, the association pushes for the legalization of recreational marijuana.

The Washington, D.C.-based association received widespread support from many people from its inception. But shortly after this organization was initially formed in 1970, its goal soon became much more difficult to achieve.

Small Victories Became Huge Challenges

The pro-marijuana factions won a series of fairly significant victories during the first few years of the 1970s, until then-President Richard Nixon put the squeeze on them.

In 1970, Roger O. Egeberg, the Assistant Secretary of Health, recommended that marijuana be temporarily placed in the restrictive Schedule I category of notorious drugs.

At the direction of Congress, Nixon appointed the bipartisan Shafer Commission, assigned to study and make recommendations regarding the drug issue.

The commission released its report on March 22, 1972, generating a controversy that soon reached a political boiling point.

The report entitled "Marihuana: A Signal of Misunderstanding" recommended that the federal government end its prohibition of the drug.

The document suggested that officials adopt methods to discourage its use, but many conservatives immediately opposed the change--which Nixon refused to implement.

The National Divide Widened

The U.S. government and many states took vastly different stances on marijuana during the remainder of the 1970s through the 1980s.

While the federal bureaucracy maintained its overly harsh, draconian anti-cannabis rules, many states gradually loosened their restrictions against the drug.

Federal anti-marijuana rules remained tight through the 1970s administrations of Republican President Gerald. R. Ford and his

186

Democrat successor, Jimmy Carter.

Meantime, conservative parents nationwide lobbied for stricter state regulations against marijuana, plus the start of programs discouraging teens from using the drug.

Partly in an effort to counteract overly harsh anti-marijuana laws, in 1974 Tom Forcade founded "High Times" magazine. Today the publication and its Website remain devoted to the legalization of cannabis.

But also during the mid-1970s, fortifying the anti-cannabis battle, powerful conservative parents established alliances with the federal Drug Enforcement Administration and the National Institute on Drug Abuse.

Conservative Tsunami Obliterated Cannabis

Hard-charging and backed by financiers with deep pockets, conservative Republicans allied with concerned parents launched the 1980s War on Drugs.

They got strong support from Republican President Ronald Reagan, arguably among the nation's most popular sitting chief executives of the 20th Century.

Riding a wave of strong public approval while heralded as "The Great Communicator," Reagan signed the Anti-Drug Abuse Act imposing mandatory sentences for the possession, use, sale and distribution of marijuana.

This overly restrictive action pounded a proverbial final nail on the political coffin of pro-marijuana advocates, at least for the foreseeable future.

The Crime Control Act of 1984 increased federal penalties for using and selling the drug; on a case-by-case basis specific penalties for each person convicted in federal court for such offenses were hinged on the amounts of narcotics involved.

Reminiscent of England's notorious Star Chamber courts of law from the 15th Century through the mid-17th Century, during the Reagan administration Congress imposed a "three strikes and you're out" rule, mandatory life sentences for repeat drug offenders. Drug kingpins faced possible death penalties under the new law.

Besides extremely dangerous narcotics such as heroin and cocaine, these worst-level drugs still included marijuana--far less lethal and destructive than alcohol.

Public Debate Intensified

Public debate regarding drugs accelerated after President George H.W. Bush made a nationally televised speech in 1989, announcing the start of a New War on Drugs.

Conservatives still embraced laws making marijuana use a serious crime, despite the findings of researchers who declared that the drug is relatively safe and even helpful.

Tragically, however, public sentiment began to change in 1996, when voters in California made theirs the first modern-era state to allow the use of marijuana for certain medical reasons.

Since then, the divide between state laws and federal regulations has been clouded as increasing numbers of states approve or consider legalizing recreational and/or medical marijuana.

Adding confusion on a nationwide basis, streams of states have approved medicinal cannabis--with rules varying widely in numerous jurisdictions.

Legalize All Drugs?

Entering the political fray, well into the 21st Century a Global Commission on Drug Policy recommended legalizing all drugs worldwide and in the United States.

Presidents George W. Bush and Barack Obama ignored the recommendations generated by a prestigious international panel of politicians and business leaders.

Besides former U.S. Secretary of State George Schulz, the panel consisted of former presidents from many countries and ex-

Federal Reserve Chairman Paul Volker.

The panel cited humanitarian and financial reasons in making its suggestion of legalizing marijuana along with other drugs.

Proclaiming the multi-decade war on drugs a dismal failure, the panel insisted that legalizing drugs would curtail violence and the rampant illicit production of narcotics.

Compounding the problem, according to the commission, taxpayers and governments get burdened with the time, cost, maintenance and development of prison systems for incarcerating drug addicts and pushers.

After extensive research on these interrelated issues, the commission said that legalizing drugs would advance its goal of bettering the "health and welfare" of mankind.

In late 2014 and early 2015, President Barack Obama commuted the sentences of hundreds of people who had been convicted of non-violent drug offenses; in many cases those crimes had involved marijuana. Spokesmen for the White House and the Attorney General said that the people had been convicted under "outdated and unfair laws." These cases had involved lengthy prison sentences for non-violent offenders. Several of these felons had been scheduled to spend the rest of their lives in prison.

Ongoing Debates Persist

For as long as humanity exists, the intense debates on these issues likely will continue because people have strong and vastly differing opinions on drugs.

Amid the continual debates and ever-changing drug laws, consumers everywhere can and should do much more to learn the "positive truth" about marijuana.

Gone are the days of ignorance such as bogus claims that cannabis makes people aggressive rapists, sexual deviants and murderers.

Instead, politicians, consumers and "average people" everywhere need to learn far more about the typical physical and mental symptoms that marijuana generates.

Upon learning that cannabis is relatively harmless when used in moderation by adults, officials should categorize this substance within a "safe and natural category."

As a natural and relatively safe substance marijuana should be legalized for adults, even if other much more dangerous drugs like heroin and cocaine remain illegal.

24
Marijuana Possession Laws

Following the lead of the United States, starting in the 1930s virtually every country worldwide enacted laws making marijuana possession illegal.

Yet to the delight of many pro-marijuana advocates, gradually during the early 2000s many countries began to decriminalize possession of small quantities of psychoactive cannabis.

Providing additional encouragement to people who like to smoke or eat psychoactive cannabis, several nations refrained from ever criminalizing marijuana possession.

Jamaica, Uruguay, and the Netherlands--all having liberal laws regulating marijuana--each lured many psychoactive cannabis users determined to avoid any threat of possible arrest for using their favorite drug.

Also, in 2013 the U.S. the federal government decided to refrain from blocking the decriminalization of marijuana in states that decided to legalize marijuana.

Severe Penalties Remain

Although anti-marijuana laws have loosed up somewhat in many jurisdictions on a sporadic basis throughout the United States, people who like using the drug should keep abreast of current regulations in jurisdictions where they live or travel.

The laws from nation-to-nation and among various states vary so significantly that every traveling marijuana user would need an "international bible of cannabis laws."

For instance, the federal government allows officials at all U.S. Indian reservations to regulate the decriminalization of cannabis.

Uruguay has even looser restrictions than Jamaica and the

Netherlands, allowing the distribution, cultivation and sale of marijuana.

Further complicating this issue on an international level, many countries have legalized cannabis when used for medical purposes.

Enforcement Efforts Vary Significantly

Complicating matters further on the domestic front, U.S. enforcement efforts vary significantly from state-to-state and among regions.

As if such paradoxical situations were not already enough to cause confusion, the federal government still strives to convict people accused of producing and distributing marijuana on a massive scale.

This confusing "domino effect" has spread worldwide, with some nations enforcing anti-marijuana laws far more aggressively than others.

Adding to this paradox, most countries have vastly diverging laws; penalties within the various jurisdictions of a single nation sometimes range from mild to severe.

All along, some countries have been steadily loosening laws for the possession of extremely small amounts--with penalties usually ranging from confiscation to small fines.

Habit-Breaking Rules

Marijuana is the world's most popular illegal drug, according to a 2013 article in "Lancet," reporting on the first international study on the use of illicit substances.

Rather than filling prisons, some nations send young occasional or perpetual users of psychoactive cannabis to mandatory drug abuse treatment programs.

Cracking down further, numerous companies including many U.S. firms require unannounced frequent or sporadic drug tests of all employees; lots of these firms fire any person discovered to have marijuana in their bloodstreams.

Some companies such as Walmart also have imposed mandatory pre-employment drug tests designed to detect marijuana and other illegal drugs.

Some countries even require the imprisonment of any person found to have cannabis in their bodies, detected when taking pre-employment drug tests.

Within East Asia and Southeast Asia, the most severe laws against marijuana use and sale carry a possible penalty of life in prison or even execution.

According to some researchers, the most restrictive cannabis laws are in France, Sweden, Indonesia, China, Turkey, Singapore, Thailand, the Philippines, Japan, and the United Arab Emirates.

Convoluted Historical Regulations

Long before becoming illegal elsewhere, marijuana served an essential role in religious ceremonies throughout some countries-- particularly India and Nepal.

Yet as previously stated, anti-marijuana laws became widespread worldwide starting in the 1930s as many nations chose to mimic the United States.

Marijuana restrictions have sporadically tightened and loosened on an international scale, particularly during the past 75 years.

At least one nation has even "tightened the screws" somewhat on marijuana, after previously having a wide-open society that freely allowed the sale and use of the drug.

Beginning on January 1, 2013, for the first time ever the Netherlands began imposing a new marijuana policy designed to combat drug-related crimes. For the first time, cannabis coffee shop owners in that nation had to monitor their customers' IDs.

According to a 2014 report by the Netherlands government, people buying cannabis there must provide IDs to prove their citizenship in that country. Additional restrictions also were imposed in that nation. Among them: Cannabis shops cannot sell alcohol; no sales are allowed to minors; marijuana cannot be sold in amounts greater than five grams in a single transaction; and each community is now responsible for the licensing of every cannabis shop within the boundaries of its jurisdiction.

Milestone Transition

In May 2013, the "New York Daily News" reported that Colorado Gov. John Hickenlooper signed laws legalizing the recreational use of marijuana in that state.

"Certainly, this industry will create jobs," the governor said. "Whether it's good for the brand of our state is still up in the air.

"But the voters passed Amendment 64 by a clear majority. That's why we're going to implement it as effectively as we possibly can."

The federal ban against marijuana officially continues, although recreational cannabis also became legal in Washington state, Alaska and other jurisdictions.

As previously mentioned, under federal regulations marijuana remains classified as a highest-level Schedule I illegal narcotic. To pro-cannabis advocates this is a critical factor, because federal law has priority over local or state laws.

This means that technically, anyone arrested by "the feds" for possessing or selling cannabis in states that have legalized the drug still face federal prosecution.

At least for now, federal enforcement remains sporadic--yet harsh and continual on a widespread scale within the continental United States.

Also, as previously mentioned, at least into mid-2015 the feds refrained from making wide-scale arrests at licensed cannabis shops in states that have legalized the drug.

Arguments for Legalization

Pro-marijuana advocates frequently have listed several arguments when campaigning for the legalization of cannabis.

Among their frequent talking points:

Tax revenues: The legalization of marijuana would open up a huge new revenue source for state and local governments, a consumer tax on the amount of product sold.

Organized crime: Legalizing marijuana is hailed as the equivalent of the end of Prohibition, a severe blow to criminals that grow, distribute and sell the drug.

Policing costs: Legalization would reduce the costs of maintaining federal and local police, according to a 2010 report from Harvard University.

Such arguments have gradually convinced many voters and consumers that legalization of the drug is a viable or even preferred option.

According to various reports, only 16 percent of Americans surveyed in 1969 supported or agreed with the concept of legalizing marijuana.

This compares with numerous surveys during the second decade of the 21st Century, when more than half of people polled wanted marijuana legalized.

Anti-Marijuana Arguments

Many law enforcement officials, families and churches have joined in a nationwide opposition to attempts to legalize marijuana for recreational use.

Often backed by conservative political organizations, these groups insist that their arguments against loosening cannabis laws are far more urgent than many people realize.

Launching political campaigns urging voters to support "No" on legalization ballots, these anti-marijuana advocates cite numerous reasons. Among them:

Youth: Legalization would make marijuana more accessible to teens, putting their brains and long-term memories in serious jeopardy throughout their lives.

Philosophies: With marijuana use spreading, young people would have fewer adult role models eager to teach them them long-term dangerous of cannabis use.

Health: Scientists lack adequate studies on the probable long-term health consequences of consistently using marijuana over extended periods.

Ambition: People using marijuana apparently think and move at a slower pace than sober individuals. Excessive widespread cannabis use might slow the economy.

Families: Anti-marijuana advocates worry about potential adverse impacts on families, particularly in instances where mothers and fathers often abuse the drug.

Counter-Arguments Emerged

The pro-marijuana crowd in Colorado insists that much has been done to address the issues voiced by anti-pot groups since recreational cannabis became legal there in 2013. People who support marijuana use in Colorado list several factors in their favor:

Teen consumption: As reported by Colorado state government officials, the use of marijuana by teenagers never increased after the drug became legal for adults.

Educational campaign: Using $2 million from marijuana sales tax revenues, the state funded an educational program teaching teenagers about the dangers of cannabis.

Decreased use: The use of marijuana by Colorado teenagers actually decreased after the state made cannabis legal for adults.

Family impacts: There apparently had been little or no significant negative impact on families due to the law change, at least according to pro-marijuana advocates.

Arguments such as these were already being echoed by pro-marijuana organizations amid subsequent cannabis legalization ballot initiatives elsewhere.

Pro-Active Action

Perhaps sensing that their actions would emerge as a model for other states, officials in Colorado took other decisive actions to limit the public appeal of marijuana.

One of the most decisive transitions came in 2012 when the Denver City Council prohibited billboard advertising that would promote businesses that sell cannabis.

The prohibitions also regulated such advertising for businesses that sell medical marijuana, particularly on billboards within 1,000 feet of schools and daycare centers.

Yet according to the "Huffington Post," pro-marijuana organizations remained divided on the advertising issue that involved First Amendment free-speech rights.

Some people had complained about or expressed their concerns regarding rampant advertising by a glut of medical marijuana shops that saturated Denver.

Additional Issues Emerged

In the initial states legalizing recreational marijuana, officials in Colorado, Washington state, Oregon and Alaska began facing issues other than cannabis use.

The wide range of potential problems or issues spanned from the growth and transportation of marijuana to licensing, taxation, security and accurate bookkeeping.

These challenges marked the emergence of a whole new set of guidelines, all underscoring the need for comprehensive, easy-to-understand regulations.

These rapidly emerging factors collectively point to the undeniable fact that marijuana rules and regulations will continue evolving for many years.

On a broad scale, the legalization of marijuana throughout the U.S. can be compared to the onset of freedom in Russia after the fall its "communist state."

Starting in the early 1990s that nation almost immediately

found itself faced with a myriad of difficult-to-regulate issues. These ranged from sudden rampant pornography to the massive, barely regulated startups of wide-scale free market businesses.

Russia's national and local officials needed well over a decade to reign in "social freedoms that had run amok," until the point where free enterprise became manageable.

Well, the same holds true here in the United States, at least within the realm of marijuana legalization. Authorities nationwide will need the time and resources to identify "what works and what fails," thereby identifying optimal ways to impose sensible rules.

Executions for Selling Marijuana

Tragically, while many U.S. states were busy loosening marijuana laws, several other countries were imposing new death-sentence rules prohibiting sales of the drug.

Historians say that within the United States no person has ever been executed by any state or the federal government for using, selling or distributing marijuana.

This has transpired on the domestic front, although U.S. federal law allows for the execution of people convicted of possessing "extraordinary amounts of the drug."

Such an amount would be "the equivalent of a forest of weed," at least 60,000 plants or at least 60,000 grams of the product-- although much safer than alcohol.

Additionally, U.S. federal law allows for the execution of people from criminal enterprises involving contraband such as marijuana, netting at least $20 million in sales.

Despite these federal regulations, the U.S. Supreme Court has ruled that treason and murder are the only crimes that can constitutionally carry the death sentence.

Executions Continue Elsewhere

Sadly, the governments of numerous Southeast Asia and East Asia countries continue to slaughter people convicted of distributing marijuana.

These draconian regulations serve as an extreme reminder that cannabis users need to remain vigilant in knowing marijuana laws--particularly when traveling.

These executions are most frequently imposed in Singapore, Thailand and the People's Republic of China. Within China, such punishment is being carried out at a "frenzied pace," according to an online Website, StopTheDrugWar.com

Many of these executions in China reportedly are timed to coincide with the United Nations International Day Against Drug Abuse and Illicit Drug Trafficking.

Also, according to several Websites, within Thailand some executions for marijuana are done on an "extra-judicial" level without trials for the defendants.

The other nations imposing death penalties, but on a less frequent level, are Indonesia, Malaysia, and the United Arab Emirates.

Per-Capita Cannabis Use

Possibly due to the imposition of death sentence for using cannabis in China, that nation has the world's lowest per-capita use of marijuana.

According to nation-to-nation surveys, a minuscule 0.03 percent of individuals older than 17 in the People's Republic of China have used the drug. This equates to a mere three out of every 1,000 adults in that nation.

These totals compare to a whopping marijuana use rate of 51.6 percent of people aged 16 to 34 in the United States. This equates to 516 out of every 1,000 people in that group; reliable estimates still are being compiled among Americans older than 34.

Authorities lack any official theory on why marijuana use is significantly different between these nations. Yet China's strict law serves as an an obvious deterrent.

Even so, some perplexing data has emerged. Only 22.6 percent of people aged 15 to 64 have used cannabis in the Netherlands, where the drug is legal for residents.

Keeping the Netherland statistics in mind, perhaps social status, education and the availability of other drugs like alcohol play key roles in determining marijuana use rates.

Annual Use of Marijuana

A diverse and varied range of public surveys taken worldwide by various public polls indicate that the U.S. has among the world's highest marijuana use rates.

In these polls people were asked numerous versions of the question, "Do you use marijuana at least once per year?" or "Have you used it within the past year?"

According these reports, 13.7 percent of people surveyed within the United States admitted to having used marijuana--a rate far higher than most industrialized countries.

Only two of those nations generate higher per-capita cannabis use, the Czech Republic at 15.2 percent and Italy at 14.6 percent.

Among nations considered to have third-world or impoverished economies, only a handful of other countries generated higher marijuana use rates than the United States. These include the African nations of Ghana at 21.5 percent, and Sierra Leone at 16.1 percent.

Significance of Data

Sociologists and experts in criminology consider the data on the per-capita use of marijuana as significant gauges into why, how and where people use the drug.

Although cannabis reigns as a natural substance generally safe when used in moderation, key roles involve the drug's availability, regulations and social acceptance.

Such data might emerge as increasingly significant in coming decades, particularly if restrictions on the drug continue to loosen in the United States.

You see, particularly through the second half of the 20th Century, many countries followed the lead of the United States in imposing marijuana restrictions.

Perhaps this occurred largely because at the time the U.S. was considered a world leader, deemed in the minds of many as "the most powerful country on earth."

Under such a mindset, the leaders of other nations likely believed that "America must be making such restrictions the right way and for important reasons, so maybe we should do this as well."

Since then, however, at least according to many political analysts, from the perception of many countries the U.S. has lost its former standing as the "greatest nation on earth."

With these key factors as a cornerstone, many fascinating questions are likely to emerge on an international scale. Namely, will other countries follow the lead of the United States in loosening marijuana laws, or will they "go their own way?"

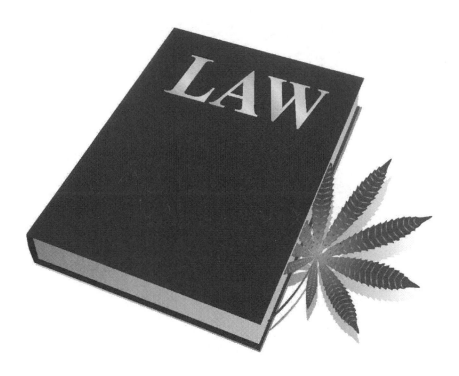

25
Marijuana Legalization Issue Reaches Boiling Point

Relentless in their efforts and vowing eventual victory, many organizations have continued their political quest to remove marijuana from the federal Schedule I list.

As stated earlier, this restriction classifies the drug as among the worst, highest-level narcotics resulting in the most severe penalties on the federal level.

This overly harsh and politically motivated restriction has failed to dampen the efforts of those who continue to insist on removing cannabis from the schedule.

In the more than 40 years since the federal Controlled Substances Act of 1972, this vigorous political battle has continued intensifying at a heated rate.

Opponents of the law still insist that marijuana fails to meet the rule's strict criteria as an extremely dangerous narcotic. Specifically, opponents want the federal government to stop controlling the drug, and to allow cannabis for medical use.

Government Stands Strong

Despite intense opposition to the law, the federal government has remained strong and steadfast in maintaining and enforcing this ill-advised restriction.

Even so, anyone who has carefully studied marijuana and its many obvious benefits should realize that the outdated federal law is overly harsh.

By maintaining this law, the federal government is essentially treating the general public as "stupid," while conveying to the masses that "we know better than you."

Indeed, the current law is based primarily on antiquated thinking and even racism that soiled the public's overall perception of the drug starting in the early 1900s.

Former President Richard Nixon seemingly embraced such a mindset for purely political reasons when signing this ill-conceived Act into law.

Since then many congressmen and senators, both Republicans and Democrats, have refrained from updating the rule--seemingly fearful of becoming perceived as weak.

The so-called "losers" here have been people who desperately need the medicinal benefits of marijuana, plus those convicted of violating these overly harsh regulations.

Political Damage Persists

Hundreds or even thousands of people remain incarcerated in federal prisons after being convicted of violating this antiquated and cruel law.

Essentially on a federal level these prisoners are being severely punished for activities now considered legal and permissible on a state and local level.

On a grand scale, these paradoxical regulations signify the ineptitude and incompetence of government in general.

Indeed, the same federal government that has harmed the nation's medical and insurance industry with Obamacare has the audacity to regulate marijuana.

Individually and collectively any politician who supports and advocates the continued listing of marijuana under Schedule I is providing a disservice to all of society.

Abolish the Federal Restriction Now

Today's elected leaders in Washington need to show the same gumption and political courage as our nation's forefathers.

Yes, now is the time for Congress with the backing of the president to remove marijuana from Schedule I, acknowledging the many benefits of using this drug.

Just as important, our politicians need to champion personal freedoms, particularly among people who refrain from causing harm to other individuals.

Rather than essentially striving to "protect society from itself," our elected leaders must do more to shield our citizens from the "Strong Arm of Government Run Amok."

Certainly, the growth, sale and distribution of marijuana must be regulated, but not to the detriment of common-sense logic that says: "This is helpful when used right."

Continue Political Efforts

The ongoing peaceful political efforts to remove marijuana from Schedule I should strengthen at an even even more rapid pace than during the past 40 years.

These strategies to overturn the rule began almost right away in 1972 thanks to the previously mentioned National Organization for the Reform of Marijuana Laws.

That effort's intense initial legal case went to the U.S. Court of Appeals in 1974, and some congressmen unsuccessfully tried to appeal the rule in 1981.

A proposal to reclassify the drug into the less-severe Schedule II category received initial bipartisan support before dying in committee.

According to the Americans for Safe Access organization, every year since then Congressman Barney Frank reintroduced similar legislation that always went nowhere.

The U.S. Drug Enforcement Administration, a federal agency that enforces drug laws, in 1986 began a two-year round of hearings on possibly rescheduling cannabis.

The next milestone came in 1988 when an administrative law judge for the agency ruled that marijuana lacks the attributes necessary for inclusion into Schedule I. Judge Francis L. Young said that natural cannabis hails as "one of the safest therapeutically active substances known to man," and he proclaimed that marijuana belongs in the less-harsh Schedule II category.

Sadly, however, a bureaucrat, DEA administrator John Lawn, overruled Young's declaration in 1988 during the final year of the conservative Reagan administration.

A U.S. federal appeals court affirmed Lawn's decision in 1994, noting the fact that doctors testifying for reclassification failed to list a single scientific study--except for in one instance.

Marijuana Advocates Refused to Back Away

Refusing to accept the overly harsh federal rule, in 1995 pro-marijuana advocates filed another petition asking the DEA to reclassify the drug.

"High Times" magazine filed the petition, but instead of using medicinal purposes as a reason, the publication stated cannabis has little potential for abuse.

The petition included documentation from a scientific study conducted from 1988 to 1994 by the National Institutes of Health.

As reported by the New York Academy of Science, that report concluded that the brain's dopamine-producing areas lack cannabinoid receptors that would cause addiction.

Essentially, this means that marijuana's psychoactive effect occurs in a different area of the brain than other illegal narcotics use to generate a high. As a result, unlike psychoactive cannabis, those drugs generate addictions; these narcotics or substances range from opiates and cocaine to cigarettes and amphetamine.

In response, a White House agency on national drug control policies asked the Institute of Medicine to review scientific evidence on cannabis' medicinal qualities. Two years later in 1997, the Institute recommended that the federal government allow marijuana for medicinal use by certain patients--yet only for short periods.

Political Games Intensified

Pro-marijuana advocates and opponents of the drug each claimed that irrefutable scientific data supported their respective positions.

According to some reports the federal documents actually refrained from recommending cannabis for medicinal use, but pro-marijuana advocates said otherwise.

Those who argue for the legalized use or rescheduling of the drug soon claimed at least one victory. In 1999, federal authorities rescheduled Marinol, the brand-name medical product derived from marijuana, from Schedule II to the less severe Schedule III.

Organizations and individuals who know that marijuana is relatively harmless had finally won at least one hard-fought victory in bringing some common sense to the rules.

Even so, in 2001 the DEA issued its final denial of the petition by John Gettman and "High Times," a decision upheld by an appeals court in 2002.

Relentless Efforts Continued

Undaunted pro-marijuana advocates spent the subsequent decade through 2012 issuing more petitions, still seeking to have the DEA reclassify the drug.

The initial petitioner in that phase, the new Coalition for Rescheduling Cannabis, won the support of medicinal marijuana users and others who joined in the legal battle.

In 2003, one year after the Coalition filed its petition, the federal agency agreed to accept the latest petition for consideration.

Adding to the legal and political firepower for pro-marijuana advocates, in 2005 in an unrelated cannabis case the U.S. Supreme Court issued a ruling favorable to Coalition's cause.

The overriding issue centered on the Gonzales vs. Raich case involving the production and use of home-grown marijuana. The court ruled that the commerce clause within the U.S. Constitution gives Congress the right to criminalize the drug, even in instances where the substance is intended for medicinal purposes.

Yet in a footnote writing for the majority decision, Justice John Paul Stevens made a brief statement giving hope to pro-marijuana advocates. Stevens proclaimed that if the scientific reports given by cannabis supporters emerge as true, such information would "cast serious doubt" on the Schedule I classification.

Justice Ruling Sought

Apparently frustrated and still seeking justice, in May 2011 the Coalition filed another motion seeking to require the DEA to finally issue a formal ruling on the 2002 petition. The agency finally denied the initial request two months later.

In issuing this oddball ruling the federal bureaucrats proved to the world once again that they make self-serving decisions--rather than considering scientific facts.

Yet who could blame them? After all, by accepting the request the agency would have eliminated one of the keystone regulations justifying that bureaucracy's existence.

Imagine the huge number of such bureaucrats and their agents who would lose their jobs if authorities adopted far more sensible anti-drug regulations.

Refusing to accept defeat, other pro-marijuana organizations and at least one politician promptly vowed to continue the political and legal fight.

In 2011, another petition with the DEA seeking to reclassify marijuana to Schedule II was filed by Washington state Governor Christine Gregoire. Rhode Island Governor Lincoln Chafee signed Gregoire's petition, which if approved would allow pharmacists nationwide to fill marijuana prescriptions issued by physicians

Heating up the issue, in late 2012 Democrat Congresswoman Diana DeGette of Colorado introduced keystone legislation. If approved, DeGette's proposed amendment to the Controlled Substances Act of 1972 would prohibit the federal government from enforcing anti-marijuana rules in states that have legalized the drug--for either medicinal or recreational use.

Meantime, adding to this paradoxical situation on a national scale, as previously mentioned, each state approves, maintains and enforces its own drug-classification schedules.

Many stories have involved highly educated, law-abiding citizens who banded together to help lead ongoing battles to legalize cannabis.

26

Important Cannabis Stories

Streams of milestone developments in recent decades have involved marijuana, almost as if peaceful rivers that eventually converge into waterfalls.

Many stories have involved highly educated, law-abiding citizens who banded together to help lead ongoing battles to legalize cannabis.

Other significant events have involved scientists who courageously started vital marijuana research, despite felony-level laws that criminalize possession of the drug.

Additional instances as recently as the 1960s have involved "everyday citizens" sentenced to many years in state prisons, merely for possessing a single joint.

The instances of "heroism" in the peaceful effort to legalize the drug are so numerous and widespread that describing all in full would be impossible. Yet several of these instances are worthy of mentioning:

The Cannabis Buyers Club: This ground-breaking facility in 1992 became the first legal medical cannabis dispensary in the United States, located in San Francisco.

Proposition 215: California voters approved this initiative, nicknamed the "Compassionate Act of 1996," thereby making their state the first to legalize medical cannabis. The law enables patients, or the caregivers of these individuals, to use prescriptions issued by doctors to purchase medical marijuana. Patients who receive approval also can grow and possess cannabis for their personal medical use. Since the law's initial enactment, state lawmakers have expanded the rules to allow such patients to collectively grow marijuana, also operating a cooperative for distribution.

Federal Enforcement in California: Particularly during the decade following the passage of Proposition 215, throughout California federal law enforcement agencies and the U.S. Attorney's Office aggressively prosecuted, raided and imposed civil injunctions on any leased property used for the production and distribution of medical cannabis. In 2008 during his initial run for president, Barack Obama promised to end DEA raids in the Golden State. The following year, U.S. Attorney General Eric Holder announced that the administration had effectively ended federal raids in California--which had continued through the administration of President George W. Bush.

Obama's Failed Promises: Despite somewhat of a victory by pro-cannabis advocates in California, President Barack Obama broke his 2008 campaign promises to decriminalize marijuana nationwide. While campaigning, Obama had promised that as president he would respect state marijuana laws. Pandering to voters but never fulfilling his vows, Obama also argued that existing federal prohibitions against the drug should be reconsidered. During the first six years of Obama's administration, 1.7 million people have been arrested nationwide for non-violent drug violations, half of them for cannabis-related offenses.

The Campaign Against Marijuana Planting: Nicknamed "CAMP," this campaign began in 1983, comprised of more than 110 California state, local and federal law enforcement agencies. Participants worked to eradicate the illegal cultivation and distribution of cannabis. Still in operation today while headed by the California Department of Justice's Bureau of Narcotic Enforcement, the many participants range from the U.S. Drug Enforcement Administration to the U.S. Forest Service, Bureau of Land Management, California State Parks and California National Guard. Despite these collective efforts, on an overall national percentage basis Golden State residents remain by far among the biggest users of illegal and medicinal marijuana.

Various California Pro-Marijuana Initiatives: During numerous elections since the 1996 passage of Proposition 215, California voters have approved numerous pro-marijuana initiatives. Among them: Proposition 36, in 2000 by a 61 percent to 39 percent margin, voters decided that qualified defendants convicted of non-violent drug possession receive probation rather than prison sentences; and with Proposition 5, in 2008 voters approved the Non-violent Offender Rehabilitation Act. It requires the state to increase funding, expand and monitor treatment and rehabilitation programs for parolees and non-violent drug offenders. The updated regulations also reduced penalties for non-violent drug offenders.

Pro-Marijuana Activist Setback: In 2010 California voters rejected Proposition 19, an initiative that would have legalized various marijuana-related activities in the state--while allowing local governments to enforce regulations. The "yes" vote for approval received only 46.5 percent. As previously stated, since then voters and legislatures in Washington state, Colorado, Oregon and Alaska have passed similar regulations. Initiatives that would legalize marijuana also were planned for several other states.

Chris Bartkowicz: This man granted an interview to a Denver local TV news crew in 2010, describing his service in Colorado as a state-licensed care-giver providing medical marijuana. Soon after the broadcast officials raided and arrested Bartkowicz on orders from DEA agent Jeffrey Sweetin. According to a report by the "New York Times," by issuing the arrest order Sweetin defied Attorney General Eric Holder's announced policy never to enforce the federal marijuana prohibition--in cases involving medicinal marijuana caregivers. According to Associated Press reports, several days after the arrest Sweetin revised his stated reason for ordering the arrest. This time Sweetin stated that Bartkowicz had allegedly provided cannabis to 12 registered patients--while possessing 12 marijuana plants for each of those individuals.

That was far more than the six plants and two ounces of the drug allowed per registered patient under state law. Colorado's attorney general protested to the DEA and Department of Justice.

Conant vs. McCaffery: In this civil case involving doctors and patients, the U.S. District Court for the Northern District of California affirmed that medicinal marijuana can be recommended by physicians--ruling that they have a right to do so.

Marijuana Business Daily: Founded in 2011, this Denver-based publication provides news of interest to the medical cannabis industry nationwide, published by Marijuana Business Media, a division of Anne Holland Ventures Inc. In 2014 the publication predicted that by 2018 the cannabis industry would grow to $8 billion, a sharp increase from an estimated $1.5 billion in 2013.

Patients Out of Time: Founded in 1995, this patients advocacy organization, nicknamed "POT," consists of nurses and other medical professionals who strive to work in cooperation with the federal government in an effort to reclassify cannabis; members want to downgrade the possession and sale of the drug from a top-level Schedule I felony.

Daktory: This operated at a warehouse in the Auckland community of New Lynn, in open defiance of New Zealand's prohibition against cannabis. Required to be over 17 years old, members paid a $5 entrance fee before openly smoking cannabis. According to news reports as recently as 2010, Daktory plans regional facilities in all major New Zealand cities. A September 2011 report on New Zealand Television said Dakta Green, the founder of Daktory, had been jailed for 23 months for operating the warehouse.

THC Ministry: Founded in 2000 in Hawaii by Roger Christie, this organization has claimed to be a religion that performs a sacrament by smoking cannabis. A federal grand jury in 2010 indicted Christie and 13 other people on allegations that they possessed and trafficked the drug, according to reports in the

"Honolulu Advertiser." Various news stories have said that the THC Ministry believes that "cultivation and enjoyment of cannabis sacrament is a fundamental right provided by God and protected by the Constitution." Since 2000 the THC Ministry has spread to at least 17 states, the United Kingdom, the Netherlands, Canada and Australia. According to several news reports, in 2013 Christie--a former G2 intelligence analyst for the U.S. Army-- pleaded guilty to two counts of failing to file income tax returns and marijuana trafficking. In 2014 a judge sentenced him to five years in federal prison, with credit for time already served in Honolulu. In early 2015 the federal case against Christie and his wife Share remained on appeal at the Ninth Circuit Court in San Francisco.

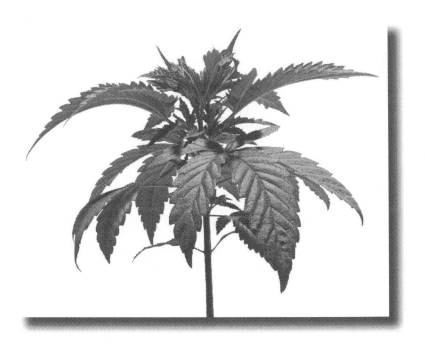

27
Hashish: The Powerful Marijuana Product

An increasingly popular product derived from marijuana called "hashish" or "hash" contains highly concentrated amounts of THC, the plant's psychoactive ingredient.

Also loaded with high concentrations of cannabinoids, hash is packed with "trichomes," comprised of stalked resin glands that have been compressed or purified.

Hashish contains extremely high concentrations of the buds and leaves that generate the calming and often peaceful high that many cannabis users enjoy.

In essence all this results in a product that enables users to get super-high, while consuming lesser quantities of total product. A single "hit" or puff from hash can make a person just as stoned as smoking standard, everyday, unmodified marijuana for an extended period.

Hashish is usually produced and sold in two forms:

Solid: The high concentrations of THC and cannabinoid are usually pressed tightly together, to form a seemingly "solid" piece of material.

Resinous: Frequently called "bubble-melt hash," this paste-like substance usually has varying degrees of pliability and hardness. Resinous hash is usually dark brown, but sometimes appears as if "see-through" in red, yellow-tan or even black colors.

The type of hashish generated hinges on the specific production process used, and the amount of leftover product that is considered unusable.

Many Specific Varieties

Many different specific, unique forms of hashish have been developed worldwide- over thousands of years, modifying or creating various varieties, subspecies or strains.

The English words of "hashish" and "hash" are derived from an ancient Arabic word that means "grass." Ironically, within the United States the term "grass" is often used as a nickname for marijuana that has not been transformed into hashish.

According to various reports, including the book "Hashish!" by Robert Connell Clark, massive hashish production accelerated in international markets during the 1960s.

Clark's book says that much of this worldwide trade began to meet the demands of U.S. "hippies," starting from Morocco, where cannabis was widely available.

Countless Generations Participated

As previously stated, historians say that hashish production began as long as 10,000 years ago. Scientists have discovered one of those ancient sites in the island nation of Taiwan off the east coast of China.

According to three pages from the diaries of Dutchman Jan Huyghen van Linschoten, in 1596 he mentioned a product called "Egyptian hashish."

A Protestant, this man called the hashish "Bangue," which he explained had been used under various names and forms in Egypt and Turkey.

The Egyptian form was called "Assis," a watery form made in paste or dough, usually eaten in five chestnut-sized pieces.

As a merchant, traveler and historian, van Linschoten wrote that Assis was used "by the common people because it is of a small price, and it is no wonder" because the product "excessively filleth the head."

Unique Consumption Methods

Rather than eating the product, many hashish users today use a variety of separate and unique methods to use this modified, highly concentrated THC--usually inhaling vapors. Among the most popular methods for using hash are:

Heated pipe: Heating up a standard pipe normally used for smoking tobacco.

Hookah: Also known as a "waterpipe" and various other names, this multi-stemmed or single instrument vaporizes flavored tobacco or hashish for smoking. Before being inhaled, the vapor or smoke passes through a water basin; these basins are often made of glass. Hookahs originated in Persia, before spreading to India and Egypt during the 823-year Ottoman Dynasty that began in 1299, before eventually entering other countries worldwide. A 2005 report by the World Health Organization concluded that smoking a hookah poses a health hazard.

Bong: Sometimes called a "waterpipe" but in this instance occasionally nicknamed with such terms as "billy," "bing" or "moof," these filtration devices are popular among cannabis smokers--and also people who like smoking tobacco or various herbal substances. Bongs are generally constructed like hookahs, but are smaller and thus much more portable. For many centuries bongs have been used throughout Africa and Southeast Asia. The word "bong" is derived from a Thai word that means a cylindrical pipe or a container that has been cut from bamboo. Some publications claim that bongs can trap heavy water-soluble particles, a filtration process that prevents those substances from entering the smoker's airways.

Vaporizer: Sometimes spelled "vaporiser," this device does what the name implies; it vaporizes cannabis or other plant-based products like tobacco. Users do this to inhale anything from marijuana to chemicals, usually mixed with plant materials. Vaporizers use numerous extraction chambers to eliminate unwanted substances. Comprised of materials ranging from metal to glass, the chambers regulate the pressure-flow of fluids. Some users collect the resulting vapors in an inflatable bag, or they inhale from a hose or pipe attached to the vaporizer. People who prefer these devices sometimes claim that when used properly this technique requires cooler temperatures than bongs and hookahs. They claim that as a result under ideal conditions vaporizers give users "a much better high." Also, partly as a result of its chamber system, at least according to numerous reports, when used to inhale marijuana, vaporizers emit fewer harmful substances than when merely smoking rolled-up marijuana "joints." An effective vaporizer might prove beneficial to people who smoke marijuana for medical purposes.

Hashish Production Processes

Marijuana buyers, harvesters and distributors use various and sometimes vastly different processes to generate and compress highly concentrated levels of THC from marijuana plants.

The primary focus almost always involves grandular hairs from the plant called "trichomes," loaded with far more cannabinoid than most other areas of cannabis.

By far the greatest concentration and number of trichomes comes from flowers of mature female marijuana plants. Although trichomes often grow on other parts of the plant, hashish producers generally focus most of their efforts on the flowers. This is because the highest THC concentrations are within the flowers or buds.

Additionally, marijuana growers often strive to produce and cross-pollinate plants in a focused effort to sharply increase the high concentration of flowers in their crops. This is done even in instances where the growers never intend to produce hashish.

The primary methods used to extract trichomes from cannabis plants are:

Mechanical: The growers, volunteers or their paid personnel use motorized tumblers or even sieve via hand using screens. Both techniques are called "dry-sifting," a process that ideally creates a powder called "dry-sift" or "kief." At this point the workers use heat to compress the powder into blocks. A pure kief results in a pliable or gooey hash. Under ideal conditions, the product contains super-high levels of THC, appearing almost transparent.

Solvents: To dissolve the desirable lipophilic resin, some manufacturers use chemical-based solvents like hexane or ethanol. After extracting highly concentrated THC, the leftover plant materials are usually put in a compost. The desirable resins are left behind when the solvents are dried off or boiled away. The resulting product is often called "oil," "honey oil," or "hash oil." Often containing essential oils and waxes, the "honey oil" is sometimes further purified into a "red oil." A vacuum distillation process does this. Technically, "honey oil" is not hashish because a sifting process extracts THC-laden trichomes.

Explosive Dangers Exist

At a disturbing and steadily increasing rate, people have been injured by explosions in various communities nationwide as they make hash at home.

These individuals called "amateur" hashish producers inadvertently spark fires and ignite explosions when using butane or other gasses to extract THC from marijuana.

These accidental explosions have become so pervasive that officials in Colorado and Washington state--where recreational marijuana had been legalized--said in 2015 that they wanted to ban amateur hash cooks from using explosive gasses including propane.

Sometimes called "concentrated marijuana," hash apparently has increased in popularity nationwide, largely thanks to this substance's ability to remain strong when mixed with food.

Much of this "explosive problem" stems from the fact that hashish is far less expensive to make at home than buying it from licensed marijuana dispensaries.

As a result of these extreme dangers, the specific and various methods of using explosive gasses to extract THC from marijuana will not be described here. Needless to say, amateurs should avoid attempting this, and doing so would be "at your own risk."

An additional extreme danger emerges when using benzene to make and process hash; as an organic chemical compound, benzene has an extremely elevated carcinogenicity. Such substances are deemed as directly involved in causing cancer. Authorities apparently lack any conclusive data on the possible percentages of hashish users who developed cancer as a likely result of using benzene.

28
Powerful
Cannabis Varieties

"They have outlawed the Number One vegetable on the planet," said the late Timothy Leary, the previously mentioned psychologist and writer who advocated psychedelic drugs.

During the height of Leary's fame from the 1960s until his death in 1996, Leary never could have sampled the many powerful cannabis varieties that exist today.

At an increasingly accelerated pace in recent decades marijuana growers worldwide have aggressively generated new and powerful varieties.

Part of this was done to meet intense consumer demand for psychoactive cannabis containing the highest-possible THC levels. This trend, in turn, created somewhat of a domino effect.

After many consumers use super-powerful marijuana products for the first time, overall they never again want "low-quality grass."

Specific Strains Emerged
Intense consumer demand motivated clandestine entrepreneurs to develop, cultivate and grow specific strains—each with a unique name and psychoactive attribute.

As previously mentioned, consumers worldwide have developed nearly 100 nicknames for marijuana. Generally, these terms ranging from "pot," "grass," and "weed" should not be confused with the specific strains specifically developed for consumers.

For many buyers and even marijuana harvesters this continual effort brings to mind a famous line from the 1993 film "Jurassic Park"--"Life finds a way."

You see, unlike most living creatures, human beings enjoy the intense and seemingly mystical powers of creativity.

Over time entrepreneurs have creatively developed unique marijuana varieties to enhance their own enjoyment of the drug, and also "out of necessity" in order to increase their profit potential.

With this clearly understood, today's consumers can choose from a variety of apparent medicinal benefits and different highs. Buyers are becoming increasingly informed about the 38 most common strains of cannabis. They are:

Acapulco Gold: This unique cannabis sativa strain famous for its gold-colored leaves originally started in Southwest Mexico. First included in the "Oxford Dictionary" in 1969, this highly coveted strain grew in what linguists described as "only in the vicinity of Acapulco." However, scientists say Acapulco gold actually grew as far south as Columbia, a country within the northern regions of South America. Within Columbia, this strain is often called "Columbian Gold." In Columbia and Southwest Mexico, Acapulco Gold has become famous for its golden-green or brownish gold leafs. According to the Oxford University Press, this strain usually costs more than greener varieties largely due to its superior potency. Publications as long ago as 1996 indicate that the "gold" term in its name refers to the strain's overall superior quality, rather than merely the increasingly famous golden tinge of its leaves. Another famous strain called "Acapulco Red," named for a reddish hue to its leaves--rather than gold--also began growing within that region. Acapulco Gold quickly became so famous during the "Hippie Generation of the 1960s" that the term was widely used in dozens of songs, publications and even subsequently in the inaugural 1975 season of "Saturday Night Live."

Afghanica: Sometimes nicknamed "Skunk," this unique strain famous for looking somewhat like a Christmas tree at full growth should never be confused with a hybrid cannabis strain called

"Afghan Kush." Botanists classify Afghanica as an extremely unique plant because it is scientifically categorized between both the separate "cannabis sativa" and the "cannabis indica" species. Scientists say this unique blending of the subspecies occurred through a process called "hybridization"--generating offspring from two plants or animals of different genres, species, varieties, or breeds. When growing wild within nature Afghanica matures rapidly with a bright green throughout summers before becoming ideal far harvesting at mid-autumn. Small, white, hairlike structures appear on the plant at maturity, loaded with super-powerful levels of THC. Upon growing to approximately 6 feet tall, the plant has an overall broad and stocky appearance accented by broad leaves crisscrossed with well-defined veins. Dense buds accentuate a lush overall canopy. The leaves occasionally develop a red or purple color when harvested in somewhat cooler conditions. Organic soil usually generates somewhat sweeter varieties. Also, in order to reach full maturity Afghanica generally requires less nutrients than most other cannabis strains. As a naturally protective measure, at maturity the leaves sometimes smell slightly like petroleum, and the buds sometimes become oily to the touch. Despite these occasionally sharp, turbulent or bitter smells, Afghanica usually has a sweet taste. More important, on a medicinal level this strain has been highly effective in treating pain or insomnia while also providing relief for stress and nausea. From the perspective of people who enjoy getting stoned, Afghanica has a relatively good THC content of just more than 20 percent. On the potential downside, however, Afghanica sometimes causes dry eyes, dry mouth and dizziness.

Alaskan Thunder-(Blank): In this instance the word "blank" is used, in order to avoid a term that some readers might consider offensive. (The actual word is a four-letter term starting with the letter F, a scatological term referring to sexual intercourse.) This strain receives relatively little attention in most scientific or cannabis-fan publications, perhaps because many people find the name highly offensive. This strain has been extremely difficult to obtain because the plant grows in the wild within the extremely remote Matanuska-Susitna Valley region of South-Central Alaska. Despite its horrific self-protective smell often described as similar to "skunk" or "cat urine," this strain has received an A-plus ranking from numerous medicinal marijuana organizations. Sometimes heralded as "one of the best strains ever," this variety often gets categorized as ideal for pain, while generating a fast and phenomenal high. Pro-marijuana advocates insist that this hails as one of the best strains for generating intense "munchies," the previously mentioned desire to eat as much as possible.

Bay 11: This award-winning medicinal marijuana strain is produced by a Los Angeles-based company founded in 2003, "Grand Daddy Purp Collective, Inc." Heralded as super-powerful, largely for its medicinal qualities, Bay 11 won the 2011 High Times Cannabis Cup competition. The annual contest held in Amsterdam was founded in 1988 by Steven Hager in conjunction with his "High Times" magazine, which has continually advocated marijuana legalization. Besides Los Angeles, Grand Daddy Purp operates California clinics in South Lake Tahoe, Santa Rosa, San Jose, Vallejo and Richmond. One of at least 17 cannabis strains sold or under development by Grand Daddy Purp, Bay 11 has been characterized as ideal for pain relief and sleep disorders. The company's many other strains range from the hybrid "Blue Dream," ideal for insomnia, anxiety, stomach pain and muscle pain, to the Silver Haze hybrid for enhancing mental focus and creativity, and the "Skunk" sativa for stress relief and appetite.

BC Bud: Primarily grown in the Canadian providence of British Columbia, this increasingly popular strain has frequently been clandestinely exported to numerous Western states-- particularly California, Oregon, Washington state, Idaho and Alaska. The growth and importation of BC Bud has become so pervasive that in 2000 the U.S. Drug Enforcement Administration declared this strain and its popularity a major problem. BC Bud became so popular while also in such intense demand that the drug became the subject of discussion in a 2007 documentary film, "The Union: The Business Behind Getting High." The intense highs generated by BC Bud are so legendary and in such intense demand that a publication of the University of Toronto Press has estimated that growth and sale of this highly coveted strain generates $6 billion yearly. Historians believe that BC Bud first evolved in the 1960s when hippies moved to British Columbia and started growing marijuana within that region's unique weather conditions ideal for cultivating marijuana. Authorities belive that much of the BC Bud is grown in chemical solutions without soil--with the primary objective as the production and consumption of marijuana buds, rather than the overall plants containing lesser amounts of THC. According to a 2004 "Time Magazine" article, officials believed that the many diverse BC Bud growers cooperated with each other in a combined effort to optimize the strain's superior high.

Black Tuna Gang: This once-famous strain technically no longer exists, first named in the 1970s after an organized crime gang that smuggled cannabis into South Florida. According to various reports, at one point during that era the gang smuggled more than 500 tons of marijuana, basing operations at least temporarily at the Fontainebleau Miami Beach Hotel. The FBI and DEA worked together to smash the ring, which never formally called itself the "Black Tuna Gang;" journalists created the name after learning that gang members identified themselves by wearing gold medallions embossed with black metal shaped like tuna.

Blue Dream: Rarely mentioned in media reports, this strain combines the Blueberry and Haze strains comprised of half sativa and half indica. The THC content reportedly is lower than many varieties, with only 15 percent to 20 percent of the psychoactive material.

Blueberry: This unique cross between the famous Highland

Thai strain sometimes called "Juicy Fruit," Blueberry also contains features of Oregon Purple Thai and Afghani male. Entrepreneurs developed this strain dominated by cannabis sativa characteristics from the late 1970s through early 1980s. According to some reports the original creator developed at least 100 unique hybrids and crosses within this strain. Unlikely Acapulco Gold, the Blueberry strain is largely known for its purple and blue coloring in both leaves and flowers. Fans insist that this strain has a blueberry taste enhanced with a fruity aroma. Best of all from the standpoint of many marijuana users, this variety has a powerful ability to generate euphoric and mellow feelings. A one-time winner of the previously mentioned High Times Cannabis Cup, Blueberry serves an ideal role in muscle relaxation, pain relief and for reducing anxiety and stress.

Charlotte's Web: Previously mentioned and produced for medical purposes, this strain lacks psychoactive attributes that generate a high. Although packed with substantial cannabidiol content, Charlotte's Web contains only 0.3 percent of psychoactive THC. This strain is famously named after a girl that has been previously mentioned, Charlotte Figi, born in 1986. The child was just five years old when her first dose of this unique marijuana strain reduced her severe epileptic seizures caused by Dravet Syndrome. According to an April 2014 issued of "Wired" magazine, six brothers developed Charlotte's Web by crossbreeding a marijuana strain with industrial hemp.

Diesel: Rarely mentioned in-depth in most cannabis publications, this strain is among those that emit a slight aroma described as similar to the smell of petroleum. At least eight subsets of the Diesel strain have been identified, including the sweet, sour and purple varieties. Among these are East Coast Sour Diesel, which--like others within this strain--have the pungent sour scent, yet with psychoactive attributes that generate mood-enhancing and uplifting highs.

G-13: Containing both sativa and indica phenotypes, the

G-13 strain was first generated from the previously mentioned Afghani variety. Crossbreeding enabled farmers to stress the female to the point that they transformed into "hermaphrodites," a biological term designating a living thing that contains both male and female features. This way, a G-13 marijuana plant contains "male flowers" that pollinate the "female flowers" on the same plant. The G-13 strain also is related to the G-14 strain available in some areas of Southern Africa. Often described as a "strong, wild variety," a daughter of the G-13 strain, the G-14 variety emits a potent fruity smell. To some extent G-13 has become an urban legend, with specifics about its development in the late 1960s and early 1970s difficult to verify. Data varies widely on the average THC content, with claims ranging from "weak" to "strong."

Haze: Reported as high in THC content and low in cannabidiol (CBD) attributes, Haze is somewhat famous for its powerful psychoactive effects. Occasionally nicknamed "amphita-weed," this strain's uplifting qualities likely become possible thanks to the plant's lengthy flowering times. Reportedly first developed in the 1970s in California and rarely seen in its pure form, Haze has many subset strains; some published reports claim that an entrepreneur, sometimes called "the Skunk man," bought this strain from the United States to Amsterdam for commercial breeding. The original developers of haze reportedly used crossbreeding in combining or mixing sativa strains from India, Thailand, Mexico and Colombia. At least 30 subset strains have been identified, ranging from Blueberry Haze to Utopia Haze.

Holland's Hope: Thanks largely to this plant's innate resistance to pests and mold, some growers reportedly prefer to harvest this indica-dominant strain outdoors. Among the first popular Dutch strains, created in the 1980s, Holland's Hope was specifically developed to endure harsh outdoor conditions. Thanks to its 100-percent indica attributes, this plant has powerful natural resistance to fungus attacks, mildew and mold.

Jack Herer: This unique and much-sought-after strain has won a whopping 11 High Times Cannabis Cup Awards. Extremely high in psychoactive attributes, this coveted strain reportedly was developed by crossbreeding the THC-rich attributes of Northern Lights No. 5, Haze and Skunk No. 1 varieties. Specifics are difficult to verify on how this crossbreeding actually occurred. Some unverified reports indicate that entrepreneurs developed Jack Herer in an effort to minimize the six-month flowering time of the powerful Haze strain. The Jack Herer strain is named in honor of a hemp proponent, the author of "The Emperor Wears No Clothes," and a longtime activist supporting the decriminalization of cannabis. Admirers of the Jack Herer strain claim this plant has excellent medicinal qualities, ideal for treating depression and stress--while also enhancing creativity, concentration and stimulating energy.

Kaia Kush: A cannabis indica hybrid hailed as one of the strongest medical marijuana strains on the international market, Kaia Kush is a cross of Super Silver Haze and OG Kush. The Kush strain hails from the Hindu Kush mountain range stretching between central Afghanistan and northern Pakistan. Medicinal professionals with expertise used crossbreeding to create Kaia Kush in 2005. Blessed with an earthy and spicy taste, it is sometimes hailed as a "soothing and enjoyable workday medication."

Kush: This strain derived from cannabis found in Afghanistan, northern Pakistan and northwestern India was a primary variety for developing the previously mentioned Kaia Kush. A British firm, GW Pharmaceuticals, has been legally licensed in England to conduct a commercial trial of Kush as a medicinal cannabis. Some reports indicate that the Kush strain, particularly OG Kush and Pink Kush are now grown in California.

Malawi Gold: Often hailed as among Africa's best sativa strains, Malawi Gold originated in the southeast Africa nation of Malawi. Called "chamba" in much of that area, Malawi Gold reportedly has been hailed by the World Bank as among the world's "best and finest" marijuana strains. Boasting highly potent psychoactive attributes, this drug has energized the Malawi tourism industry as visitors stream to the region to get high. This strain has become so increasingly popular that it has been listed among the three Big Cs: Chamba (Malawi Gold); Chambo (Talapi fish); and Chombe (tea). The Malawi Gold strain has many medicinal, religious and recreational uses. The "BNL Times" reports that a vast majority of the Malawi Gold crop is exported. Various reports indicate that this strain has been used to treat snake bites, malaria, fevers, dysentery, and exposure to anthrax.

Morning Star: Botanists have not yet identified the origins of this cross of sativa and indica cannabis. Users insist that the potent Morning Star strain has fast-acting attributes ideal for generating upbeat positive feelings. These sensations are accompanied by an enjoyable but mellow "buzzing body high." Some medical experts insist that Morning Star serves as an ideal remedy in treating migraines, insomnia, anorexia, anxiety and pain. With a 24-percent THC content, this plant has light green buds featuring long orange pistils. The flavors when burned range from hash and spice, to skunk and sour fruit.

Nederwiet: This strain from the Netherlands labeled with the Dutch word for "skunk" in the 1980s originally had been called "the poor man's weed" with extremely low THC content of just 8 percent. Determined to correct this "problem," according to published reports, in the 1990s students at the Dutch University of Agriculture successfully upgraded the strain to the point where the THC content reached 25 percent. Several publications since then have listed the average THC content at around 20 percent. This significant boost in psychoactive potency has sharply increased the popularity of Nederwiet, hailed as twice as strong as most cannabis strains available in the European Union.

New York City Diesel: Although generating what users describe as an excellent high, this sativa-dominant strain has been described as lacking the psychoactive power of its parent strains--

Sour Diesel mixed with Afghan indica.

Northern Lights: A small plant at only 4 feet to 5 feet in height at maturity, this high-yielding, indica-dominant strain is considered potent. Boasting a spicy, sweet taste with a pungently sweet aroma, the plant gained fame at harvest festivals while also winning the 1990 High Times Cannabis Cup. Eventually with five subset strains, Northern Lights was originally bred in Seattle, Washington. The original Northern Lights strain evolved into 11 distinct plants; these are named Northern Lights numbers one through 11.

Panama Red: Famed for its potency, this pure cultivar of cannabis sativa, also called "Panamanian Red," first became popular in the 1960s and 1970s. The unique characteristics of this marijuana plant generate an extremely high THC content, rather than the unique Panamanian weather, according to a 1971 report issued by the U.S. Department of Health, Education and Welfare. In 2004 researchers at Auburn University grew Panama Red in the diverse climates of northern New Hampshire, Panama, and various climates of the canal zone--generating high THC content in each instance. Sociologists say the plant's name originated from the nation where its cultivation began, plus a reddish color in the leaves. Much of the clandestine cultivation occurred in the Pearl Islands, a group of about 200 islands in the Pacific--most about 30 miles from the Panama coast. Cultivation of Panama Red in that nation faded during the 1970s and 1980s, replaced by illegal cocaine trafficking.

Purple: This subset of the indica-dominant strain is generated by seasonal temperature changes. The green usually overpowers its many colors, including orange, red, and the most highly coveted color of purple. The purple is derived from water-soluble vacuolar Anthocyanin pigments. Scientists have identified five subsets of purple cannabis: Mendocino "Purps;" the previously mentioned Afghan Kush; Purple Urkel; Grand Daddy Purp; and Grape Ape.

Purple Dragon: This highly potent strain of cannabis sativa, sometimes called "Apalala," was created when entrepreneurs cross-bred two extremely powerful and popular strains--BC Bud and Purple Haze.

Purple Haze: Dutch seed breeders reportedly developed this cannabis strain famous in part for its massive swaths of deep color. Featuring a fantastic potency graced with an abundance of white trichomes, this unique strain is thought by some researchers to be extinct--presently regarded as having seemingly mythical status.

Purple Kush: Heralded as one of the most potent strains of marijuana, although having hints of sativa, this plant primarily has indica characteristics. Some people mistakenly believe that all Purple Kush have leaves of that color; botanists say that the leaves of any cannabis strain can emit purple if temperatures cool during flowering. When used via inhaling, the smoke contains an extremely high THC level that emits a distinctive, unmistakably flowery taste. Depending on specific strategies used in curing and drying processes, the high when smoked can last two hours, according to some published reports. Although cannabis users seem to lack universal agreement on which strain is best, many people reportedly consider Purple Kush as a powerful relaxant that generates a fairly long-lasting and pleasant high. Standing only 2 to 3 feet high when fully grown indoors, Purple Kush are significantly smaller than most strains--which typically reach an average of about 6 feet.

Quebec Gold: This highly potent strain is found primarily within the Quebec community of Canada. With a full-bodied flavor and a sweet citrus smell, the sativa characteristics of Quebec Gold generate heavy psychoactive effects. Embossed with dense buds and a resin often described as "exceptional," this marijuana is sometimes used to produce a deep and powerful hashish that is almost black. The term "Quebec Gold" is sometimes used as street talk throughout that community when referring to any powerful cannabis bought and sold in the community. Some users claim that Quebec Gold is just as good or even better than the famous previously mentioned BC Bud strain, also produced in Canada. According to some unverified stories and publications, law enforcement officials consider Quebec Gold as the U.S. East Coast's equivalent to BC Bud--which is commonly imported to West Coast states.

Sharkberry Cream: This strain receives relatively little media attention, although proclaimed winner of the 2012 High Times Cannabis Cup in the "import" category. Pro-marijuana advocates describe Sharkberry Cream as a cross between the little-known Great White Shark and Blueberry strains. Besides producing a fantastic high, Sharkberry Cream reportedly has intensive psychedelic qualities.

Skunk: Although considered among the most famous and highly coveted cannabis strains, this plant actually generates a smell similar to that of a skunk. Used by the plant as a protective measure from predators, the odor when emitted by this strain supposedly generates little concern from its most ardent fans. Yet largely due to the offensive smell, when harvested by entrepreneurs this plant is usually cultivated indoors in an effort to avoid detection by law enforcement. As a hybrid of cannabis sativa and cannabis indica, the various subsets of Skunk and its primary strain all have unique characteristics. Although highly popular among recreational cannabis users for many years, Skunk and its subsets have become a focus of interest among medical experts. Scientists reportedly have been studying the effectiveness of Skunk in treating many difficult-to-treat ailments. Even so, some physicians and cannabis users worry that Skunk might potentially have more negative side effects than other marijuana strains. According to a post at "Web MD," Skunk might be more dangerous because the strain contains far more THC content than any CBD capable of counteracting the extreme highs. The numerous possible negative side effects range from anxiety and paranoia to short-term memory loss. At least 18 subsets have been identified, with names ranging from Amnesia Haze to Island Sweet Skunk. The previously mentioned Northern Lights strain reportedly is a Skunk subset.

Tangerine Dream: A cross of Neville's A5 Haze and the previously mentioned G-13, this sativa-dominated strain generates the cerebral experience typically generated by sativa-- plus a calming sense of relaxation typically produced by indica. Although proponents of Tangerine Dream apparently fail to list scientific data to back their claims, they reportedly say that this strain is highly effective in relieving depression, stress, nausea and anxiety. Some reports claim without backing up their declaration that Tangerine Dream boasts a mind-boggling THC content of 25 percent. Speckled with orange and red hairs, at maturity the plant has large, tightly bonded buds.

Te Puke Thunder: This rare strain reportedly was found in the early 1970s on New Zealand's North Island coast, a region called "Te Puke, Bay of Plenty." This strain reportedly has much larger buds than most marijuana plants, thereby increasing its potency. Some cannabis users consider Te Puke Thunder among the most potent and long-lasting strains. Fans of Te Puke Thunder credit the Northern New Zealand climate, considered ideal for growing marijuana. The term for this strain should not be confused with a "party pill" that has been legalized in that nation for experiencing a "legal high." Pro-marijuana advocates complain that the pill's name causes undue confusion, partly because the pharmaceutical lacks materials from this plant.

Thai Stick: Popular in the late 1960s through the 1970s, this is made by skewering buds from seedless marijuana onto stems. Sometimes this is done by creating "rasta hair," formed when using a string to secure Thai stick buds onto bamboo. Unlike most pure marijuana products, however, in some instances the producers from Thailand also dipped the Thai sticks into opium--the primary ingredient for heroin, morphine and other extremely dangerous opiate-based drugs. Particularly during the 1960s, this clandestine-generated attribute increased the reputation of Thai Sticks in the West. At the time this concoction lacked the psychoactive power of super-potent marijuana strains that are commonly grown and distributed now in the 21st Century. Not all Thai Sticks were laced with opiate-based materials. Overall these strains were far superior to those found in the West during the 1960s. Until then, over many generations harvesters in Thailand typically used only seeds from their best plants. Thai Sticks temporarily increased in popularity when smuggled to U.S. Troops fighting in the Vietnam War.

Tom Cruise Purple: The world-famous actor Tom Cruise has publicly disavowed any connection with--and proclaims that he does not condone the use of--this notorious strain that coincidentally bears his name. Sold via select cannabis clubs throughout California, this highly potent strain is sometimes marketed in packages that feature a photo taken of the actor as he laughed. The product became a media sensation by 2008, a frequent subject of late-night talk show hosts, radio commentators and political analysts on TV. This unique strain emerged as far from a laughing matter to anti-marijuana groups that claim the "Tom Cruise" plant generates an extreme high accompanied by "Hallucinogenic properties," according to an April 2008 story in the "Philadelphia Daily News." Despite any objections that the actor's fans might have, the Tom Cruise Purple strain is legally sold in licensed medical cannabis stores in California.

White Widow: Somewhat notoriously famous for its extremely high potency and white trichomes, this strain was developed in the Netherlands--before winning the 1995 High Times Cannabis Cup Award. Like most cannabis strains, this generates the hunger called the "munchies," but also a super-relaxed feeling. Typically a 60-percent indica and 40-percent sativa, White Widow often creates a mood enhancement that reportedly motivates new users to engage in activities that they typically would refrain from trying. Embossed with an almost snowy appearance due to its white crystal-covered buds, this strain is sometimes grown in

Amsterdam with THC contents averaging 20 percent. While this compact plant usually reaches medium height, the buds typically have only a few amber-colored hairs. The plant's distinctive white comes from a unique crystalline resin.

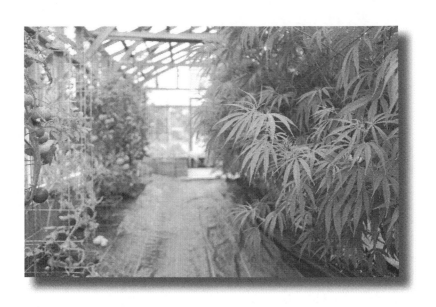

29
Cannabis
Cultivation Methods

Although infrequent exceptions occur, the marijuana cultivation process is typically done in an effort to enhance and increase the "high."

For this reason, most marijuana "farmers" concentrate on developing and growing cannabis plants that have many buds containing huge amounts of THC.

Before and during the growth and harvesting process, each grower must determine which genus or family of the particular cannabis species is involved.

This becomes critical for many factors, primarily because most strains typically are "dioecious," meaning that individual plants have either male or female characteristics.

In addition, some individual strains of marijuana plants have both male and female characteristics, giving them an ability to self-populate or "reproduce themselves."

There are four species within the cannabis family of "Cannabaceae," characterized by botanists as a "small family of plants." Within this overall classification, scientists have identified 170 specific species; many of these are trees and "herbaceous" or herb plants that lack the ability of cannabis to generate psychoactive THC.

Growth Requirements

Certain conditions are necessary in order for marijuana to grow and thrive, both in the wild and when cultivated. Among them:

Temperatures: Optimal daytime temperatures averaging 75 degrees to 86 degrees Fahrenheit. Temperatures higher than 88 degrees tend to decrease psychoactive potency.

Light: The light can either be natural when grown outdoors or artificial for indoor cultivation. When artificial light is used many growers prefer to keep the crop under light about 20 hours daily. Some growers debate the importance of any "dark period."

Nutrients: When grown in soils, the basic nutrients of nitrogen, phosphorous and potassium are necessary. Some growers cautiously include nutrients by adding fertilizers to the soils. The nutrient benefits and requirements vary during specific growth stages; more nitrogen than the other nutrients is necessary during the vegetative stage, and the plants need more potassium during the critical flowering stage. Some growers recommend the secondary nutrients of sulfur, magnesium and calcium. Each strain or variety of cannabis has its own unique nutrient requirements, so many growers determine the best solutions via a "trial-and-error" process.

pH levels: On the pH scale, optimal results often occur when soils and even fertilizers are in the slightly acidic range of 5.9 to 6.5.

Water: Many factors determine the amount and frequency of necessary water, with results dependent on everything from the plants' ages to the stage of growth and size. Marijuana plants can die from too much watering.

Unique Growth Stages

Like all plant species, each strain or variety of cannabis has its own unique development phase. Among these primary features:

Germination: This initial phase can take as little as 12 hours to eight days, a necessary point where seeds sprout and roots form. Ideal levels of light, dark, moisture and warmth trigger this initial phase, activating metabolic processes that start an expansion inside the seed, the growth of an embryo. Ideally prior to this point the seed had been placed in a suitable place, suitable for the roots to emerge and grow downward. Then, if all goes as planned, two initial embryonic leaves emerge from the soil in a search for necessary light. At this point the seedling stage begins if the newborn plant has been able to push away any remains of the seed shell.

Seedling Phase: Generally lasting from one to four weeks, this milestone period marks a phase when the new plant is most vulnerable to excessively harsh weather, too much sunlight, or inadequate or even excessive amounts of water. For these reasons, during the seedling phase many growers strive for: adequate rather than excessive soil moisture; light intensity at medium to high levels; and moderate humidity. To minimize heat, during this period many indoor growers use T5 fluorescent or compact fluorescent lights. Higher-power lights likely would damage the seedlings by drying out root systems. Identifiable sex characteristics usually appear in four to six weeks; some growers intensify lights to accelerate each plant's declaration of its sex. Growers remove the male plants once this happens, because the desired females produce the greatest quantities of THC from their buds. Yet this initial effort reportedly can increase the necessary time for the plants to reach maturity. Some growers argue that the strategy occasionally decreases potency, while others disagree.

Vegetative Phase: When growing indoors, this stage can last from one to two months. The time involved hings on light and nutrients, coupled with the particular cannabis strain involved. As the sex reveals itself, the roots naturally spread like those of most plants in search of nutrients and water. Due to careful crossbreeding, some growers have developed plants that actually omit the vegetative phase; instead, such plants transition straight from a seedling to a pre-flowering plant. Normally for cannabis in its natural condition, the beginning of the vegetative phase commences at the point where the plant has seven distinctive leaves. At this precise juncture, an eighth leaf can barely be seen emerging from the growth tip's center. Throughout the vegetative phase, the plant's primary objective becomes growing the roots, stems and leaves. This phase emerges as critically important to people who want to eventually get high from the plant, because the desired potency and density of THC generated by eventual flowers or buds hinges on a strong root system. Size is an excellent indicator of sex, with females typically reaching less height than males; females usually have more leaves than males in their flowering areas and atop the plants. While careful to provide warmth and cool periods for the plants to achieve optimal health, to accelerate growth during this phase many marijuana farmers also provide their indoor cannabis crops with 18 hours to 24 hours of daily light. Also, particularly during the vegetative phase many growers strive to "train" their plants to grow shorter and with more density. Many diverse yet interlinking factors come to play in determining necessary growth times, everything from how much space is available to flower sizes and the number of plants.

Vegetative Phase Techniques: During the vegetative phase some growers use specific techniques in efforts to accelerate growth and enhance potency. The specific tactic depends on the harvesters' personal preferences or requirements imposed by their associates. These methods can include: topping, the removal of the top of the dominant central stem, thereby striving to accelerate growth in the remainder of the plant; pinching, this intentionally damages structural or vascular cells by firmly pinching--rather than removing--the dominant central stem in an effort to accelerate growth; and LST'ing, a "low-stress training" process sometimes called "super-cropping," manipulating the plants' growth by tying and bending branches into a preferred shape.

Pre-Flowering Phase: During this phase sometimes called "the stretch," typically lasting from one day to two weeks, most indoor growers set light and darkness to separate and equal 2-hour periods. Most plants increase dramatically in size during this essential phase, sometimes doubling in overall mass or even achieving substantially more volume. This sudden and extensive growth signifies that the plant is ready to flower.

Flowering Phase: Achieving the ultimate goal of producing THC-laden buds, the flowering phase typically occurs from six to

22 weeks after seedling begins. Dubbed "miraculous" by many cannabis lovers, within this stage the males produce panicles, little grape-shaped, ball-like flower clusters. The flowering occurs within diminishing light in most cannabis strains, which sense the coming onset of winter as daylight diminishes. To capture wind-blown pollen produced by males, a sticky white resin appears in the form of trichomes or glands on females that have not been pollinated by males. This urgent tactic by females to repopulate actually serves as a God's-send to cannabis users who yearn to get high; the greatest amounts of THC and CBD (Cannabidiol) are derived from resin-producing trichomes. Before this essential stage, many cannabis farmers prefer to eliminate males; *females that have been successfully pollinated produce less than half of their trichome potential.* Also, cannabis plants that fail to produce seeds are often deemed the best, considered far more potent and superior to seed-producing females. Growers face a proverbial balancing act, as they strive to manage a paradoxical situation. Decreasing the amount of light per-day accelerates flowering but decreases yield. Conversely, maintaining ample daily light for many months delays the eventual flowering process, but increases overall THC production.

Other Flowering Phase Considerations: Some growers reportedly strive to maintain exactly 12 hours of daily light in order to maintain a perfect balance. An unknown percentage of indoor marijuana producers continually "toy with" or change the hours of lighting in efforts to maximize results. Growing marijuana outdoors generates other unique challenges, particularly the ideal time for planting. Operators of some outdoor cannabis farms use black plastic to cover the plants for 12 hours daily. The strain involved becomes an important consideration because each has a unique propensity to flower at certain times. The potential for success becomes even more challenging when considering the fact that sunlight inhibits the hormones needed for flowers--by far the most coveted part of the plant.

Outdoor Growing: Many experienced marijuana growers reportedly claim that numerous cannabis strains grow best outdoors. While hundreds of strains exist, most growing outdoors requires ample sunlight during the vegetative phase, plus nutrient-rich soil. Within warmer regions relatively close to the Equator, germination or planting typically begins in the late spring or early summer. This is necessary to generate proper growth in time for harvesting, usually in the late summer or early autumn. These growers often called "outdoor cultivators," have different preferences on the types of cannabis plants or strains that they harvest. Many outdoor cultivators insist on growing indica-dominant plants that achieve "short stature," grow fast and generate high yields. Conversely, other outdoor farmers prefer cultivating sativa because that generates a "much better and stronger high," emitting less odor and responding generally well to sunlight. Outdoor harvesters unable to grow marijuana on their own properties often work "guerrilla-style," planting their crops in remote, difficult-to-reach outdoor settings like cliffs or small clearings in forests. Guerrilla farmers rarely visit their crops during the growth season to avoid being seen or arrested by authorities. Compounding these problems, some clandestine marijuana farms become the target of thieves. At least according to numerous unconfirmed and unverified reports, some outdoor harvesters set booby traps to protect their secretive marijuana farms. Numerous people who advocate the legalization of medical and recreational marijuana intentionally throw or plant cannabis seeds in wildland areas. These unorganized participants in "Operation Overgrow" strive to enable cannabis to grow wildly, sporadically and naturally throughout nature like a "natural weed."

Indoor Cannabis Cultivation

The indoor cultivation of marijuana generates many unique challenges or tasks other than those previously mentioned. Among the numerous benefits and disadvantages:

Control: Harvesters have complete control of everything from the soil to lighting times and watering.

Expense: Growing marijuana indoors is generally considered much more expensive.

Faster: These farmers can accelerate growth by leaving the lights on 24 hours daily during the vegetative phase.

Risk: Harvesters have less risk of detection by authorities.

Techniques: Harvesters can control oxygen, light, humidity, and watering, rather than exposing their plants to unpredictable and potentially harsh weather.

Lighting Requirements

When determining light, indoor harvesters must consider the unique needs of specific strains, coupled with the amount of available space and ventilation methods.

Many growers apparently use timers to turn lights off and on, everything set at pre-designated intervals. Most plants grow in the full spectrum of light, while some still manage to thrive under a single light spectra.

Various unscientific tests reportedly have been conducted to determine whether cannabis harvested indoors grows better when using high pressure sodium lamps, metal halide lamps, or a combination of them.

An undetermined number of growers reportedly claim that metal halide lamps generate optimal results. Other observers insist there is no difference.

While opinions differ sharply, numerous published reports indicate certain types of lamps might be best for specific growth phases:

Metal Halide: These lamps are sometimes deemed ideal during the vegetative phase, generating a stockier and shorter plant while inhibiting the elongation of cells, thereby decreasing the distance between leaves.

High-pressure Sodium Lamps: These lamps supposedly work

the best at producing ultraviolet radiation, thus increasing the abundance of THC-laden psychoactive flowers. For this reason, amid their pre-timed growing season some indoor harvesters stop using metal halide lamps and start using sodium lamps; this transition begins after the vegetative phase and as the flowering phase starts.

These factors likely have become less important in recent years for some indoor harvesters. Advancements in LED technology have enabled growers to control and set their desired nanometer range within the full light spectrum.

Even so, according to intermittent and sporadic non-scientific published reports, the use of LED lights when harvesting cannabis is still considered experimental.

Other Lighting Factors

Eager to optimize growth times and maximize THC, some industrious indoor harvesters use reflectors in order to use all of the available light emitted by their lamps.

This way these entrepreneurs strive to ensure that their entire crop receives equal amounts of the vital light for optimal growth and to maximize psychoactive results.

These techniques are considered so essential that some harvesters even install slightly concave canopies to reflect light, at an optimal distance from its source.

Additionally, some indoor growers also maximize the wattage in order to boost or control light levels, often set at maximum. Extensive calculations are sometimes used, factors such as the crop's the total square footage.

Just as important, at least from the perspective of some indoor harvesters, reflective materials must be installed on every wall of grow rooms.

Atmospheric Controls

New technology has enabled indoor marijuana harvesters to carefully control the growing environment, managing everything from humidity to temperatures.

While carefully maintaining specific temperatures within ideal ranges, these growers also strive to limit potentially harmful carbon dioxide levels.

Besides maintaining adequate light and nutrients, some of these ventures need air filtration systems, partly to eliminate excess odors emitted by certain strains.

Sending most of this aroma outside might tend to generate suspicion, potentially motivating neighbors to notify authorities. To avoid such problems, some growers push air from their harvesting rooms through carbon filters.

Additionally, rather than recirculating, some indoor cannabis farmers send the air outside; this is only done after first using filters to eliminate odors.

Whatever type of air circulation system is used, growers must minimize or prevent the excessive buildup of ozone concentrations in their gardens. Excessive ozone levels are harmful to all life.

Cannabis Farmers: Dedication Required

Marijuana farmers need high levels of dedication, commitment and competence, the same personal attributes necessary for most entrepreneurs to achieve success in almost any type of business. Yet such characteristics fail to obliterate the difficult-to-avoid reality that growing marijuana is illegal in most jurisdictions and still a high-level felony under U.S. federal law.

Particularly within the United States, harvesters of cannabis grown indoors or outdoors need to take measures to block or eliminate the possibility of being detected. Their challenge seems even more dauting when considering the fact that these ventures face the additional challenge of mastering many complex or interlinking techniques.

Many indoor marijuana growers choose to start out small when initially launching their ventures. Lots of these individuals realize the need for extensive harvesting experience before attempting to master the many complex requirements on a broad scale.

Largely as a result, when starting such ventures many first-time indoor marijuana growers initially dedicate a closet or single room for their ventures.

Later, when and if such initial efforts emerge as successful, some growers increase their "garden areas" to several rooms or entire basements.

After enjoying a sudden surge of incoming cash, numerous growers quickly expand or move their indoor garden areas to small, mid-size or large warehouses. Yet extreme dangers often emerge when this happens, primarily a sharp increase in the possibility of detection by the U.S. Drug Enforcement Administration.

Excessive greed within this wide-open industry has led some growers onto a pathway toward lengthy sentences in federal penitentiaries.

For this reason, a huge percentage of indoor and outdoor marijuana harvesters strive to "operate under the proverbial radar screen," generating just enough cash to make a healthy living-- while also careful to avoid attracting unwanted attention.

Popularity of Industry Surges

According to numerous published reports, indoor cannabis farming has significantly increased in popularity since the 21st Century began.

Some sociologists, economists and criminologists say that a likely reason for this trend hinges on a substantial increase in information regarding the best techniques.

Intricate details cover everything from step-by-step instructions to equipment and seeds.

On an individual and collective basis, these interlinking factors have quickly become so widespread that harvesters have been able to purchase and maintain pre-designed, pre-built, fully-equipped "grow houses" dedicated to growing marijuana.

Largely as a result, high-quality psychoactive cannabis has rapidly become increasingly available to consumers nationwide.

Utility Costs Become Security Issue

Excessive or relatively high electric utility costs have increasingly become a security issue for new and even experienced indoor cannabis growers.

With steadily increasing proficiency, some utility companies have started working in cooperation with law enforcement agencies to pinpoint large grow houses.

Authorities often look for sudden surges in power usage at a home, or strive to detect attempts to steal electricity by bypassing meters.

Determined to remain at least "one step ahead of the law," some environmentally conscious growers install gas-, diesel-, or solar-powered electricity production systems. These tactics sometimes "pay for themselves," generating ample energy for huge crops.

Growers who are unwilling or unable to install power generators often use other strategies to minimize electricity use. These tactics typically include watching less TV, keeping lights off in non-garden rooms, using low-watt light bulbs, buying energy efficient household appliances, and similar efforts.

Ozone and Smell Issues

The previously mentioned issues of ozone buildup and smell have become an increasing concern.

Chronic users and big-time growers of cannabis sometimes become so accustomed to the odors that they fail to sense what the bodies of many non-marijuana users would detect right away.

This danger becomes exacerbated by the fact that air scrubbers or filters for eliminating the smells sometimes cause a dangerous buildup of ozone indoors.

Besides endangering the plants, excessive ozone can impose a serious health risk on anyone living or working inside a home or apartment used to grow cannabis.

To side-step this paradoxical problem, some indoor marijuana harvesters firmly seal or shut windows, while also using ample quantities of air fresheners.

As a precaution, growers sometimes maintain their gardens in difficult-to-detect areas of the home such as attics or basements. An additional strategy sometimes involves selecting cannabis strains that emit less odor.

Other Dangers Emerge

Numerous other potential dangers also frequently emerge, such as a sharply increased risk of fire from faulty wiring, hazardous fixtures and improper sockets.

The potential for such dangers accelerates even more when indoor growers buy and maintain relatively cheap and old houses for their ventures.

Overloaded circuit breakers sometimes spark electrical fires at such ill-advised grow houses, posing danger to anyone inside and to the occupants of neighboring homes.

Dangers multiply due to the possibility of old, damaged or inadequate wires prone to melt and spark fires as the result of excessive electricity consumption.

As a result, some growers strive for the appearance of natural indoor lighting, used only while harvesters are at the residence.

Another common strategy involves refraining from the use of intricate, expensive and power-sucking grow lamps that might increase suspicion and danger.

Loose Lips Sink Ships

A famous phrase used often during World War I and World War II still holds true for today's marijuana growers: "Loose Lips Sink Ships."

Telling too many people, or just a single person, about a grow-house location can lead to detection, arrest, conviction and imprisonment.

For this reason, some cannabis growers prefer to work alone without mentioning the endeavor to anyone.

When selling the product they strive to work only with known buyers--preferably a trusted friend who deals in bulk.

By dealing with as few people as possible, marijuana growers sharply decrease the possibility of detection. But even then there is no guarantee of avoiding arrest.

Just like with almost everything in life, "there is always a risk."

Housing Damage Occurs

As if all these many potential pitfalls were not already enough to generate significant concern, many homes are significantly damaged when used for harvesting marijuana. These buildings are called "grow-houses."

By remodifying homes for their indoor marijuana gardens, some growers make structural changes that violate various electrical, natural gas and building codes.

Structural damage sometimes occurs as a result of these modifications. Besides increasing overall dangers, these building violations raise concerns or pose problems when the harvester eventually tries to sell the home.

Some of the worst structural damage occurs when growers drill gaping holes in walls and floors to increase ventilation. Problems worsen when doing such "stupid things" as disconnecting furnace filters.

On the positive side, such tactics sometimes replicate natural outdoor-type of atmospheric conditions--thereby enhancing all growth phases when harvesting indoors.

Even so, when using a grow room or grow house--particularly over extended periods--toxic mold and moisture can build to extremely dangerous levels.

Amateurs Leave Tell-Tale Signs

Amateurs or shoddy growers sometimes unknowingly create tell-tale signs eventually leading to their capture.

A typical case here involves a grow house that generally seems to lack any such clues, at least when the grow house is seen at first glance from outside.

Even when that happens, however, lots of growers still generate suspicion. Common"goofs" usually entail things like avoiding neighbors, using indoor heat systems that melt snow near the house, and posting unnecessary "beware of dog" signs.

According to reports and stories in 2009-2010 issues of the "Toronto Star," real estate agent John Trac unwittingly left many such tale-tell signs as the mastermind of 54 rented houses used as "marijuana grown ops." He was convicted and imprisoned.

According to a report by CBS News, the problem has became so pervasive that when remodeling or "flipping" homes for profit, some building contractors and their work crews have discovered that the houses were previously used as marijuana grow-ops.

In some communities police who raid grow houses must notify city officials of the problem. The current homeowners or subsequent buyers are required to fix the structural violations before the residence can be occupied or legally sold.

30
Curing, Drying and Harvesting

The many intricate and necessary techniques for growing marijuana are just part of the total work involved.

After the plants have successfully been grown in the desired way--or even when the product becomes substandard--lots of other chores become necessary.

At this point numerous important factors come to play; everything depends on the strain, overall crop quality and the specific type of product desired. Among common preparation or harvesting methods:

Cloning: Growers never allow flowers to appear on cannabis plants that are intended for "cloning," used primarily for the cultivation of future crops.

Hemp: When this is intended for use as a fiber, the plant must be harvested before any flowers appear.

Seeds: Only fully developed plants are used, primarily gleaned from buds as they begin to deteriorate.

Smoking: Most of the time plants intended for use as smoking products are typically harvested when a white, clear, or reddish brown appears on at least two-thirds of the pistils.

General Criteria Necessary for Desired Results

In almost every instance, no matter what the desired end-product, harvesting involves the necessary and vital processes of drying and curing.

Ideally, when curing the grower strives to generate an even distribution of moisture throughout the product.

When drying, the buds are left in a relatively dry and dark

place; curing is relatively similar, except that the buds are kept in a dark place inside sealed bags.

Some growers reportedly strive to vary their drying and curing times, such as 12- or 24-hour stretches for drying, while 6-hour periods are always used for curing.

These processes are continually repeated for three- or four-day periods until the product is deemed "ready."

For all this to begin, the cannabis buds must first be declared as fully ripe, a condition that generally occurs when the white pistils turn light to mid-red, orange, or even dark yellow.

Simultaneously, in order to also be declared as fully ripe, a milky white or clear appearance must emerge on the plant's trichomes; these biological structures also can start looking amber-red. Some growers consider a clear appearance as underdeveloped.

The Drying Process

Rather than turning up the heat to excessive levels, in most instances the drying process usually occurs at normal room temperatures of about 60 to 70 degrees Fahrenheit.

Extreme care and close attention to detail is vital during this stage, because heat above 70 degrees evaporates molecules necessary for a psychoactive effect.

Coupled with the size and density of buds, humidity plays a key factor in determining the total time needed for drying--usually two days to a few weeks.

Besides the urgent need to control temperature, growers also need to pay close attention to humidity levels when drying. For best results, humidity should remain within the 45 percent to 55 percent range throughout the drying process.

Humidity levels below or above that range can generate negative results.

When humidity stays below 45 percent during most or all of the drying process, the product dries too fast; such an unwanted or unintentional technique prevents the plant from reaching its full psychoactive potential. Compounding the problems, drying too fast can block the conversion of chlorophyll, thereby generating a less-than-desired taste. This failure also can generate a smoke deemed harsh or unpleasant to inhale.

Just as problematic, drying in humidity above 55 percent poses a risk of mold or mildew that causes health problems, while also compromising psychoactive potential.

Specialized Drying Tactics and Preferences
To the disappointment of many growers, there is no one-size-fits-all method for generating the best possible results from the cannabis drying process.

Harvesters have a variety of preferences or techniques during this phase; most strategies focus on enhancing psychoactive effects. Among common tactics:

Preservation: Cannabinoid generally remains well preserved amid environments with well-maintained temperatures.

Hanging: Enable flowers to remain on the plant by using natural internal fluids, hanging the flowers by their stalks.

Natural plants: Some growers insist that an ideal non-sticky object from stems that have been cut subsequently generate excellent future plants.

Ensure drying: Easily being able to snap stems at the middle after removing roots indicates that the plant has been sufficiently dried.

Darkness: Always dry in a dark place because light tends to deteriorate resins containing the vital THC psychoactive attributes.

Never Underestimate the Odors
For the most part, even novices generally consider the drying process as relatively safe and difficult to "do wrong." The most formidable challenges involve successful techniques and monitoring throughout the "grow" process. Yet many indoor harvesters underestimate the massive scale of odors produced

by moving, cropping and hanging the plants in order to initiate drying.

Part of the problem occurs because by this point many growers--particularly novices--have become somewhat, or even completely, desensitized to the odors. These aromas often are strong enough to attract unwanted attention, particularly within communities or region where marijuana growing is illegal.

Much of the time the odors become apparent to anyone within the general vicinity, in some cases even several houses away. The danger of possible detection intensifies in certain weather conditions including intense, moderate or even light wind.

A Common strategy for avoiding such situations includes shutting off and blocking ventilation systems. Yet some ventilation remains critical so that the harvesters can breathe healthy air, rather than inhaling pungent aromas that might sicken them.

To side-step or handle this problem, some growers use upper-level ventilation systems such as chimneys and roofs during drying.

Specialized Curing Strategies

Marijuana harvesters pay close attention to tactics used in the curing process, largely to enhance or improve the taste and smoothness of smoke.

Sometimes they use airtight canning jars for packing--but not compressing--marijuana that has already been dried. Continual diligence becomes necessary, checking to ensure that the product remains dry without re-moistening.

Growers eventually tighten the jars, but only after the product has been completely dried, usually after at least several days. Thereafter the jars are opened briefly about once every week.

The overall curing process is usually completed within about two weeks, although total times can vary depending of several factors. Everything hinges on each crop's overall quality.

Some growers prefer to take up to six months for curing, while others completely avoid this overall process. For the most part curing is largely done to enhance smoking, making the use of the crop as enjoyable as possible--thereby enticing the consumer to subsequently purchase more of the same product.

Additionally, in some instances harvesters attempt a unique process called "water curing," a strategy often deemed useful for plants considered of lower quality. This is done by watering at ample levels right to the point of harvest, partly in an effort to flush away harmful chemicals that had been used to feed the plants.

Ideally, this flushing process also rids the crop of certain resins, pigments, sugars and proteins that might "make the weed un-smokable."

Whether water curing reduces the overall THC-to-weight ratio remains a matter of dispute. Complicating matters, some growers insist that this strategy fails to work better than standard curing methods.

Tinctures Gain Attention

Using scientific knowledge to their advantage, some marijuana growers and distributors appreciate the fact that THC is soluble in alcohol.

Thanks to this unique characteristic, some industrious harvesters use ethanol to extract cannabinoids from marijuana plants. The result becomes an edible product although this extraction process usually takes longer than other methods.

These are formed into "tinctures," in broad terms defined as a liquid and alcoholic extract from a plant. When using cannabis buds, leaves and stems, the resulting tincture can be smoked, mixed with foods or eaten straight.

Some cannabis smokers enjoy THC in a clandestine or guerrilla mode, by dipping cigarettes into these tinctures. Then these users openly smoke their THC-laced tobacco in public for a highly enjoyable "hidden high."

Yet care is needed, because THC disappears from the liquid when coming into direct contact with flames, at least according to some published reports. To circumvent such problems, some smokers use straws to inhale vapors from heated tinctures.

Hash Oil Extracts

The production of hash oil extracts should never be confused with the production of hashish, details already described in a previous section.

Marijuana product manufacturers sometimes use solvents to generate liquid hash oil, which preferably has a relatively high THC content. In many instances the solvents contain one or more alcohol-based substances such as toluene or hexane, ethanol, butane or isopropyl alcohol.

These entrepreneurs use a vacuum or evaporation to remove soluble resins from plant particulates that had been filtered out by the solvents. This sometimes results in the desired high THC content; the purest THC usually is generated by using butane, which often extracts lower amounts of undesirable solubles like cannabinoids and proteins.

The various solvents other than butane are likely to generate more of these unwanted substances, resulting in less-than-pure THC content.

In an effort to prevent so-called impurities from the resulting hash oil, some producers freeze plant matter before beginning the extraction process.

Brick Weed

A typical or seldom-used cannabis packaging and curing process involves using a hydraulic press to compact the entire plant into a brick that contains the stems buds and seeds.

The result called "brick weed" gets a relatively low overall rating from experienced marijuana users because this product usually contains a low THC content.

While less potent, brick weed also lacks the mysterious or pleasant taste and aroma that many marijuana users demand and crave.

Immediately before this stage manufacturers either avoid the bud drying process, or they never attempt the compacting stage.

Much of the world's brick weed production occurs in countries or regions that produce massive quantities of marijuana, particularly Mexico and Paraguay.

Important Pest Control Advice

Many experienced marijuana growers strongly recommend avoiding the use of dangerous chemicals or pesticides when trying to control pests that attack the plant.

Everyone who grows marijuana outdoors and indoors invariably experience pest issues. Yet tragically, harvesters sometimes recklessly or unwittingly use toxic chemical pesticides that pose extreme danger to people, the plants and the environment.

To prevent such problems, experienced and even some novice growers strongly recommend using only pesticides labeled as "safe to use on food crops." Among pesticide substances described as causing little or no harm:

Azadirachtin: Non-toxic, biodegradable and classified as a natural pesticide, this often is easier to locate and less expensive than many other non-toxic insecticides.

Pyrethrins: High-production costs usually make this difficult-to-find insecticide more expensive, although heralded as effective and organic.

Neem Oil: This vegetable-based oil is produced by pressing the seeds and fruits of neem, an evergreen tree scientifically called "Azadirachta indica." Relatively inexpensive and found at major stores like Wal-Mart, this is ideal for cannabis plants, plus fruits and vegetables; Neem oil serves a variety of useful purposes as a fungicide, insecticide and miticide.

Pests that invade cannabis crops grown indoors are usually unwittingly carried inside by people and household pets. Efforts to exterminate such pests indoors often fail if the invaders repopulate to advance stages before insecticide use begins.

Advanced Cannabis Cultivation Methods

Seasoned and experienced cannabis growers use various high-tech or improved methods in their farming, along with many of the techniques already mentioned.

Besides increasing potency, these various systems try to boost overall crop size while in many instances also accelerating growth rates. Among these methods:

Training: Often done in conjunction with trellising, harvesters "train" plants to grow in certain shapes and sizes; this helps maximize efficiency, especially indoors. Many unique training and trellising methods were developed by producers of Marinol, the marijuana-derived drug legally distributed by U.S. pharmacies.

Fertilizers: These involve home-grown or organic methods, developed to optimize plant health and THC, while environmentally safe.

Growth base: With increasing frequency, some harvesters choose air-based or water-based platforms for growing. These can entail "hydroponics" that use mineral and nutrient solutions in water, or "aeroponics," the process of growing plants from an air or mist environment while using water to transmit nutrients.

Some scientists credit the use of these various techniques with enabling entrepreneurs to increase the overall number of unique cannabis strains in recent decades. Some of these potent new strains include the previously mentioned NYC Diesel, Afghan Kush and Northern Lights.

Advancements in Internet technology have been credited with making many of these changes possible as cannabis growers share vital information worldwide.

"Screen of Green" Techniques

Particularly since the beginning of the 21st Century, the "Screen of Green" method has emerged an increasingly popular way to increase crop yields and potency.

Cannabis farmers harvest only colas of the plants, usually grown with a hydroponic media. Growers place the plants in individual containers, geometrically arranged in patterns or specific places to maximize growth efficiency.

This way the entrepreneurs manage the growth rate and placements of vital THC-laden flowers and other essential plant materials, while also regulating the atmosphere and light levels.

Particularly when done on a massive or industrial-size scale, the sea of green method--sometimes called SOG--has proven helpful to commercial cultivators of large cannabis crops.

Besides minimizing the vegetative phase, this method enables growers to place plants closer to lights--while also carefully managing the distribution of light.

SCReen of Green

Similar in many ways to the standard "sea of green" process, the SCReen of Green or SCROG method enables harvesters to train the plants.

Like sea of green, SCROG enables harvesters to enhance the bud effect of each plant, thereby maximizing the overall harvest--all done while using only a limited number of plants.

This fairly ingenious method involves basic, simple technology.

In many instances SCROG involves affixing a chicken wire in a horizontal position directly over the growing area. This makes plant tips grow to the same level.

Largely as a result, when using strategically arranged lighting, all buds receive equal light levels. This becomes important because when done correctly the flowers grow through the chicken wire--giving them vital light during the rapid growth of THC.

For optimal results, when using the SCROG method harvesters

strive to keep the plants in the vegetative state until the screen is from 70 percent to 80 percent full. Prior to flowering and when the plant tips reach 3 or 4 inches above the wire, harvesters bend or pull them downward--placing the tips under the wire.

Timing and placement emerge as vital factors, while success hinges on a serious "balancing act" by growers. Harvesters strive to prevent the buds from becoming too crowded, while simultaneously trying to achieve a bountiful harvest.

Important Genetic Considerations

As if all these various techniques were not already challenging enough, harvesters also face important decisions involving the plants' genetics and gender.

The genetics issue sometimes becomes formidable as harvesters look for preferred, high-yielding strains featuring desired characteristics.

Since overall growth time and costs emerge as major factors, some harvesters perform intricate calculations on every watt spent per month--thereby determining the specific crop yield per gram.

Like the operators of almost every business, many harvesters like to know beforehand the specific projected "return on investment" for each crop or strain.

When making critical decisions on which strains to grow and how much to farm, harvesters must consider numerous interlinking and essential factors.

The many important characteristics to ponder range from overall yield and potency to pest resistance, trichome density, time to flowering, aroma and the specific strain's overall popularity among consumers.

Strains that "Auto-flower"

Besides the many considerations already mentioned, with increased frequency in recent years harvesters have needed to consider strains that automatically flower--whatever gender is involved.

This relatively new challenge involves "auto-flowering" strains that grow to maturity, significantly faster than the vast majority of most natural marijuana strains.

When using "auto-flowering seeds," harvesters cultivate plants that rapidly progress through a short vegetative period that sometimes takes two to three weeks from the time of initial germination. By comparison, most natural strains when grown in the wild or even indoors can take from three to six months to start flowering at maturity.

The flowering of plants derived from auto-flowering seeds depends on age, rather than the season, time of year or the ratio of daily light and darkness. Lighting ratios needed for full maturity can vary greatly, unlike specific light time required for the optimal growth of standard psychoactive cannabis.

The first documented type of auto-flowering cannabis seed to reach the marketplace was Lowryder Number 1, a hybrid between Northern Lights Number 2 and William's Wonder--sometimes labeled with the scientific name, "Cannabis ruderalis."

Since the introduction of Lowryder Number 1, harvesters have meticulously spent many years developing numerous auto-flowering strains. These have led to "super auto-flowers," many producing seeds that grow up to 2 meters with significant yields.

The Desired Seeds--Feminine

Despite the advent of auto-flowering, many harvesters prefer "feminized seeds" that result in females; this gender that produces by far the greatest amounts of flowers and buds packed with high THC concentrations.

However, a unique challenge has remained, especially involving wild or natural cannabis, because most marijuana plants refrain from declaring their gender until flowering time.

Adding to this formidable task, as previously mentioned,

female plants that have not been fertilized by males produce by far the greatest levels of psychoactive attributes.

This task becomes doubly challenging for harvesters. They know that plants in the wild thrive thanks to the desirable trait called the "instability of gender."

Amazingly, Mother Nature prefers instability or "unpredictability" within the wild, where reproduction hails as the most urgent goal of all plants.

Methods of Feminized Seed Production

Entrepreneurial and highly creative, through the past several decades harvesters working alone or together have devised numerous ways to produce feminized seeds.

This has emerged as critical to the overall vibrancy and efficiency of the overall cannabis harvesting industry, at the corporate level and in clandestine operations.

The basic methods require commitment and often laborious efforts. Among them:

Cloning: This entails using parts of "known mature females" to grow new feminine plants loaded with THC-laden flowers. Clones retain their parent plant's gender throughout life.

Rodelization: Going well past the normal or scheduled harvest time, harvesters allow non-pollinated females to live longer than would normally be scheduled. This triggers hermaphrodite or "self-populating" characteristics in the females; these environmental stresses sometimes generate pollen-bearing male flowers, even on females. Plants sometimes do this naturally in an effort to continue their genetic line.

Colloidal Silver Solutions: To enhance or promote the growth of feminized seeds, harvesters spray this natural solution on selected areas or even on the entire plant--particularly if trying to produce large amounts of seeds. Upon receiving such treatments at least three times weekly, most plants become "intersex" within two weeks. Four weeks after the spraying starts most cannabis plants produce viable pollen.

Gibberellic Acid: Extremely expensive and challenging to obtain, this natural substance found in limited amounts in plants and fungi is generally considered more effective than colloidal silver. Scientists have created an industrial method of creating gibberellic acid at a relatively high cost.

Preferred Results Achieved

Most harvesters seem to believe that all the previously mentioned methods for feminizing seeds are successful.

The primary goal in each instance is to put the plants under certain types of stresses that trigger genes regulating hermaphroditism. Then, in their view, the seeds invariably adopt the desired characteristics, no matter what strategy was used.

Yet this assumption is largely incorrect.

Genes from the parental plants pass to subsequent generations. This occurs whether or not genes have been stressed enough to generate hermaphroditism.

All along, most harvesters lack the type of selective breeding needed to generate the onset of female flowering, at a point before male flowering occurs.

Increasing the Vigor of Plants

To create hybrid plants, harvesters sometimes cross two strains of cannabis.

This becomes desirable because hybrids contain a unique and beneficial characteristic called "hybrid vigor."

Particularly if all goes well and as planned in the cross-breeding process, the hybrid grows faster, stronger and healthier than its predecessors.

Yet problems can occur, particularly when and if harvesters crossbreed strains that have biological characteristics unsuitable for mixing or mating.

As a result, seasoned marijuana harvesters often suggest that all growers use extreme caution when contemplating or undergoing any cross-breeding attempts.

Wide-Scale Cloning

Some cannabis harvesters clone their crops on a massive scale, in order to replicate previous successes or to accelerate overall growth.

As briefly mentioned earlier, cloning typically involves cutting part of a cannabis plant, usually at a lateral branch or even the main stem.

The cut-off plant parts can then be used to generate their own roots, thereby retaining specific characteristics of the original plant.

Ideally, these cuts or clones are done from a known female plant, thereby increasing the potential and propensity for dense, THC-rich buds and flowers.

When successful, this typically happens fast. Most of the time new roots develop in as little as five days, or as long as three weeks.

One of the most common methods involves water cloning, a strategy used by many people over thousands of years in diverse cultures for several types of crops.

Basic Cloning Strategies

Through a trial-and-error process, harvesters have developed numerous cloning techniques designed to help ensure success and to simplify the process. Among tasks:

Leaves: When cutting from the main stem, remove at least the bottom two-thirds of leaves from the cut-off part of the plant before planting it to generate roots.

Roots: To prevent fungal infections, and also to promote root growth, apply a root hormone or auxin to the cut-off part before planting.

Planting site: Plant the cut-off part, usually called a "cutting," in an area surrounded by air. Besides the previously mentioned water- and air-based planting bases, some harvesters plant their cuttings in rich soils, or substances like rock wool, peat moss, oasis foam, perlite, compost or a combination of them.

Humidity: As previously stated, elevated humidity generally tends to slow the transpiration rate. This would decrease the important ability of cannabis leaves to lose moisture. Such a condition could prevent the plant from fully drying. This condition in turn sometimes attracts dangerous mold. As a result, advanced harvesters control humidity while also keeping temperatures low enough to promote healthy growth.

Transfer: Once the roots finally form in the initial site such as water, air or soil, harvesters transfer the cuttings to their permanent growing place.

Essential Summary

In essence, as seen from the many numerous examples already given, successfully growing high-quality, thriving marijuana plants involves far more than merely planting seeds.

Knowing these basics can help consumers ask sellers the right questions.

Rather than try to identify a seller's source, strive to learn specifics about the "product" that they're distributing. Ask questions like "What is the strain?" and "What is the potency?"

Because they want to make a sale, most distributors are likely to proclaim "this is fantastic weed"--even if that's untrue.

More specifically, however, try to casually ask sellers if they know the strain of cannabis, the estimate percentage of THC, and details about any unique side effects.

Knowing the strain and potency often becomes extremely important to people who need medicinal cannabis.

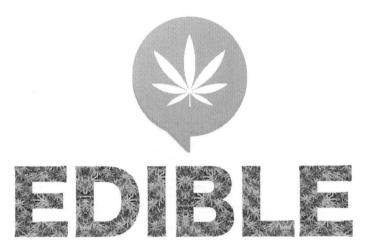

31
Cannabis Foods Abound

Many people worldwide prefer to eat cannabis baked or cooked within foods, rather than smoking or inhaling the drug as marijuana or hashish.

A wide variety of other foods for baking marijuana include cookies, cupcakes and brownies.

Unlike the instant high achieved from smoking or inhaling cannabis, the psychoactive experience usually begins one or two hours after eating the drug.

Some marijuana users say that the high lasts much longer when eating, sometimes as long as four to six hours, far longer than the mere two-hour high from smoking.

Eating psychoactive cannabis also minimizes or eliminates the potential risks to the lungs generated by smoking or inhaling. Scientists say the risks of lung cancer from smoking cannabis is unknown; a huge percentage of people who smoke marijuana also use tobacco--a factor that makes any reliable comparisons difficult.

Streams of Marijuana Food Recipes

Marijuana users from many cultures have steadily and independently developed a unique nomenclature, a huge variety of words to describe their preferred cannabis foods.

The various slang terms describing recipes range from edibles and hash, to fortified, evolved, spiked, super skunk, medicated, fabricated and many more.

When broken down to its basic form, the THC ingredient

in cannabis that enables people to get high is a hydrophobic oil insoluble in water. Interestingly, however, TCH also is soluble in alcohol and oil or fat lipids.

Thus, alcohol, oils or fats must first be used to extract this substance from cannabis; this is done to ensure that the high-producing THC remains present and potent after baking. The desired "high" fails to become possible without this critical process.

For this happen, any one of two possible strategies can be used:

Sufficient heating: Increase temperatures for extended periods.

Dehydration: Extract all moisture from marijuana's most abundant cannabinoid, "Tetrahydrocannabinolic acid." This is a biosynthetic precursor of THC.

Amateur or professional chefs or bakers need to use great care when preparing marijuana for baking. As a purified powder, THC becomes unstable when in the presence of oxygen, heat, acids or light.

Luckily, the vast majority of cannabis-preparation methods for baking never isolate THC into its purest powder form.

Ancient Fine-Tuned Recipes

Thanks to ancient recipes developed in India, scientists realize that for thousands of years people have known about the oil-solubility of marijuana.

Merely boiling cannabis to make beverages like tea fails to sufficiently extract THC in order for the drink to generate a super high. Using marijuana to make this beverage sometimes generates a low-grade high, particularly when the ingredients contain ample amounts of good-quality resins at the outside of the plant.

Heat-softened resins containing at least some THC float atop the beverage, but only thanks to varying degrees of luck and skill by these tea lovers.

Far better than water, within India the preferred liquid for making THC drinks is milk because it contains electrolytes, proteins and fats. For thousands of years people in India have successfully made a THC-rich, milk-based beverage called "bhang." Flowers and buds from female cannabis plants are the primary ingredient.

Drinking and getting high from bhang is a common practice in Nepal and India, particularly during Hindu festivals. These ceremonies usually involve large groups of men who collectively use mortar and pestle to process leaves and buds; they grind the materials into a paste.

This mixture is added to milk, spices and "ghee," a class of clarified butter commonly used for medicine and religious purposes in India, Pakistan, Afghanistan and other countries throughout that region.

After the mixing process ends, the men transform the liquid into a heavy drink called "thandai," sometimes inaccurately called "bhang lassi" or "bhang thandai."

People throughout these cultures sometimes mix bhang with sugar and ghee to make purple halva, and sometimes little chewy, peppery balls called "golee."

Besides getting stoned, people throughout India sometimes use bhang for medicinal purposes. Targeted ailments include appetite or digestive problems, sunstroke, fever, dysentery, and lisping.

Experiencing a "Better High"

Some cannabis users and publications contend that eating properly prepared cannabis foods generates a far better high than smoking the drug.

A 2004 story in the "Sao Paulo Medical Journal" said that eating cannabis generates a superior high because the liver produces a unique active metabolite, "11-OH-THC." Reportedly more powerful than THC, the metabolite easily crosses the blood-brain barrier.

A 2009 article in "Clinical Chemistry" said that THC concentrations in the body are lower when eaten than smoked. The report concluded that eating generates a higher 11-OH-THC to standard THC ratio, resulting in the better highs.

Additionally, according to the National Organization for the Reform of Marijuana Laws, the 11-OH-THC is eventually metabolized into the non-psychoactive 11-nor-9-carboxy-THC. This likely plays an essential role in some of the primary medicinal effects of cannabis, particularly as an anti-inflammatory and an analgesic.

Whether this high is better remains a matter of debate. In any case, the psychoactive effect when eating cannabis takes longer to begin because the THC must first be absorbed through the digestive tract.

Amateur and professional chefs cooking cannabis products also need skills involving the management of THCA, contained in cannabis and an acid within the carboxylic group. In order for THC to become psychoactive, substances within the carboxyl group including THCA must first be removed.

In order to optimize the ratios between THC and THCA, researchers recommend cooking for 27 minutes at 251 degrees Fahrenheit.

The "Oil" Cooking Methods

Some chefs preparing cannabis foods prefer using a method that involves "marijuana oils," sometimes called "cannaoils." Infused with cannabinoids, these cooking oil-based products are produced by extracting certain chemical constituents from marijuana.

Various methods are used to prepare these oils, a process that must include activating a chemical process called "decarboxylation." When this chemical reaction occurs carboxylic acids are removed in a process that releases carbon dioxide--a colorless and odorless gas vital to all plant life.

This chemical reaction must occur before or during the extraction of oil, in order for the resulting liquid to ultimately have psychoactive attributes. A study described in 2011 by the "Journal of Molecular Structure" identified the ideal heating and time needed to optimize psychoactive THC during decarboxylation at 230 degrees Fahrenheit for 110 minutes.

Using any cooking oil, the resulting substance must be solvated in a lipid solvent after finishing this chemical conversion. Vigorously mix the oil with the plant material for at least five minutes to 10 minutes.

Depending on personal preference, chefs can then strain the oily mixture, while also using heated oil. Some preparers prefer using double boilers to keep the temperature at a near-constant 212 degrees Fahrenheit, the boiling point of water.

Pushing the temperature above 279 degrees Fahrenheit generates the risk of vaporizing compounds out of the mixture. Of equal importance is the fact that heating at below 195 degrees Fahrenheit for less than 24 hours invariably fails to adequately generate the necessary chemical conversions, according to the "Journal of Chromatography."

The "Butter" Cooking Methods

Rather than oils, some strategies concentrate on butter-based preparation and cooking methods. Common slang terms used to describe these substances range from "marijuana butter" and "butterjuana," to "cannabutter" and "Magical Butter."

Under all these various names the resulting product has been infused with cannabis. Chefs heat butter, resin or herbal cannabis, allowing fats to remove the cannabinoids.

Rather than using double boilers, a more complicated process sometimes involves funnels, tea strainers or cheesecloth, and slow cookers. Depending on recipes, cooking times can vary significantly--as long as 24 hours and as fast as 15 minutes.

Temperatures and cooking times sometimes vary, with the duration sometimes extended if heat is lowered.

Creating Cannabis Liqueurs

People preferring or wanting to try "cannabis liqueurs" take advantage of the fact that cannabis is soluble in alcohol. And as previously mentioned, cannabis must be mixed with substances that marijuana is soluble with, in order to extract THC; only this way can "weed food" preparers activate psychoactive attributes that enable people to get high.

Besides merely mixing marijuana with brandy and rum, this can emerge as an ideal way to add THC-laced beverages to recipes for a variety of foods.

When preparing cannabis-laden liqueurs, some chefs use portions of cannabis plants that are usually not involved in preparing marijuana for smoking.

Rather than buds and flowers loaded with THC, when preparing cannabis liquors many chefs use "left-over" parts of the plant such as stems or leaves. This is done even though those sections of the plants usually contain only small amounts of THC.

Some preparers use high-proof, grain-based alcohol, creating a "Green Dragon" beverage made from potent alcohols like Ever-Clear.

One of the most popular liquor-based cannabis drink concoctions is called "Creme de Gras," translated to mean "cream of fat" and a play on the English word "grass." Some users prefer to mix this flavored liquor with coffee.

Stupendous Hashish Cookies

The notorious "hashish cookie" sometimes gets the credit or blame for a sense of euphoria, happiness and peacefulness.

These snacks contain hashish, high concentrations of the psychoactive-generating THC ingredient derived from cannabis.

Some lovers of this snack call them "Alice B. Toklas Cookies," honoring a famed author. Toklas published her recipe for "Haschich Fudge" in the "Alice B. Toklas Cookbook," her 1954 memoir that became a literary sensation.

Particularly popular in the Netherlands, "Space cookies" is another common name for certain baked goods including cookies, brownies and muffins that all contain marijuana. Until psychoactive psilocybin mushrooms were banned in 2008 in the Netherlands, some bakers in that nation sprinkled them as a frosting atop space cookies.

Baked in many countries, hashish cookies are similar to standard cannabis cookies, except much more powerful at generating highs.

Cannabis Foods Became Popular Worldwide

Some bakers also use hashish in cakes, roll the drug into ball-shaped donuts, or bake these ingredients into brownies.

Experienced users call the sensation created by baked goods containing hashish as a "high head," an overall bodily and motion sensation of feeling light-weight. Some users prefer this rather than risking the health hazards of smoking hash.

Additionally, some "stoners" also like taking these snacks to parties or locations where marijuana smoking is banned or discouraged.

Most baked foods containing cannabis or hash look like "regular" foods lacking the drug, except an occasional greenish tinge, and sometimes a slight odor.

Stories involving or featuring cannabis-laced baked food have been featured in many mainstream movies and TV shows since the 1960s. Among the most popular of these was "I Love You, Alice B. Toklas," a 1968 movie starring Peter Sellers. His character embraces the free-spirited hippie culture and cannabis-laden brownies, abandoning the confines of so-called mainstream life.

During the last half of the 20th Century, Mary Jane Rathbun, a medical cannabis activist, became widely known as "Brownie Mary."

A 1999 article in "The Independent" said Rathbun had illegally baked cannabis brownies while working as a volunteer at San

Francisco General Hospital, where she sneaked the foods to AIDS patients. According to a 1993 article in the "Chicago Tribune," the City of San Francisco eventually gave Rathbun permission to give the brownies to people with the disease. She also lobbied for passage of voter initiatives to legalize medical cannabis.

32
Cannabis Advocacy Organizations

Numerous non-profit groups work in the United States, and sometimes in other countries, in educational and political efforts to increase public awareness about the safety of marijuana. Some of these organizations strive to legalize cannabis for recreational and/or medicinal uses. Among the most influential are:

Veterans for Medical Cannabis Access: This Virginia-based non-profit organization founded in 2007, strives to protect the rights of U.S. military veterans who want access to marijuana for medicinal purposes. The organization wants to enable veterans to have a right to discuss medical cannabis with their doctors, eliminating any risk of reprisal.

Drug Policy Alliance: Founded in 2000, this New York City-based non-profit organization has a primary goal of ending the federal government's "war on drugs." Details: DrugPolicy.org

Marijuana Policy Project: Founded in 1999, this Washington, D.C.-based non-profit project is the largest organization dedicated to reforming the federal government's policy on cannabis. Details: MPP.org

Multidisciplinary Association for Psychedelic Studies: Briefly mentioned earlier, founded in 1986 and nicknamed "MAPS," this non-profit educational and research organization works to develop psychedelics and marijuana into legal prescription drugs. Details: MAPS.org

Students for Sensible Drug Policy: Founded in 1998, this Washington, D.C.-based International non-profit advocacy strives to change attitudes and drug policies, drug abuse, drug use and marijuana prohibition. Besides the United States, it serves numerous countries and continents including Mexico, Africa, Australia, Canada, Ireland and the United Kingdom. Details: SSDP.org

Drug War-Rant: Founded by Peter Guither, an assistant dean in the College of Fine Arts at Illinois State University, the name of this organization is a play on the word "warrant." The organization's Website provides a bulletin board-style system including a blog and other features, while also claiming that the federal government's "war on drugs" has actually worsened crime and terrorism. Details: DrugWarRant.com

National Organization for the Reform of Marijuana Laws: Briefly mentioned earlier, this Washington, D.C.-based organization founded in 1970--nicknamed "NORML"--strives to legalize non-medicinal marijuana in the United States. Details: Norml.org

Marijuana Anonymous: Formed in 1989, this non-profit organization is based on the 12-step recovery program used by an unaffiliated system, Alcoholics Anonymous. This program strives to help people achieve their common desire to abstain from marijuana. Details: Marijuana-Anonymous.org

American Alliance for Medical Cannabis: Founded in 2001, while advocating clinical research, this organization works with educators, clergy, caregivers, health professional and communities to promote legal access to medical cannabis. Details: LetFreedomGrow.org

American Medical Marijuana Association: Founded online in 2000, this Fort Bragg, California-based volunteer organization strives to protect and promote law reforms to guarantee and legalize access to medical marijuana. A primary objective is to protect the previously mentioned California Proposition 215. Details: AmericanMarijuana.org

Americans for Safe Access: This Washington, D.C.-based membership organization founded in 2002 works to ensure that consumers and scientists have safe and legal access to cannabis for therapeutic uses and research. Policy makers, medical professionals, attorneys, and patients receive medical information and training from the organization. Details: SafeAccessNow.org

Coalition for Rescheduling Cannabis: Briefly mentioned earlier, this organization founded in 2002 strives to legally remove marijuana from Schedule I. The organization is a coalition of at least nine organizations including Patients Out of Time and "High Times" magazine. This organization apparently has no centralized Website.

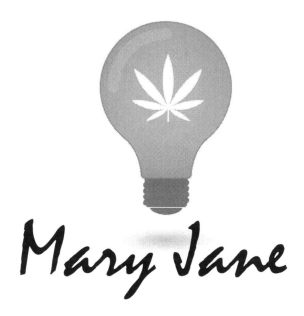

Mary Jane

33
Common Names for Marijuana

Sociologists list many hundreds of names used for marijuana. The names are so numerous that there are far too many to list in full in this publication. Yet for your convenience some of the most common are listed here:

Ashes
Aunt Mary
Baby Bang
Bammy
Blanket
Blunt
Bo-Bo
Baby Bhang
Bobo Bash
Bomber
Boom
Broccoli
Cheeba
Chronic
Cripple
Daga
Dinkie Dow
Dope
Ganja
Gasper
Giggle Smoke

Good Giggles
Goog Butt
Grass
Hash
Herb
Hot Stick
Jay
Joy Smoke
Joy Stick
Mary Jane
Pot
Reefer
Roach
Skunk
Weed

Marijuana laced with some variety of narcotic
Amp Joint
Dust
Dusting

Marijuana and Heroin
Atom Bomb
A-Bomb
Brown
Canade
Woola
Woolie
Woo-Woo

Marijuana and PCP
Ace
Bohd
Chips
Frios
Zoom

Marijuana and LSD
Beast
LBJ

Marijuana and Crack
Buda
Butter
Crack Baby
Fry Daddy
Geek
Juice Joint

Marijuana and Cocaine
Banano
Basuco
Bush
Chase
Cocktail
Cocoa Puff
Hooter
Jim Jones
Lace

Marijuana and Alcohol
Herb and Al

Slang Terms for Marijuana Use and Abuse
Blast
Blow
Blowing Smoke
Blow a Stick
Boot a Gong
Airhead (marijuana user)
Bite One's Lips
Bogart
Hi the Hay
Burn One
Fire it up
Get a gauge up
Get the Wind
Fly Mexican Airlines
Mow the grass
Tea party
Toke
Torch Up

My Clinic's Vastly Superior Survival Rate

The five-year survival rate of advanced Stage IV cancer patients treated at my clinic is nearly 33 times better than the national average in my current five-year study.

On a nationwide basis only a dismal 2.1 percent of all such patients survive after being treated by mainstream oncologists who deliver high-dose standard chemo.

By comparison, results at my Century Wellness clinic reflect a 5-year survival rate of more than 67 percent among such patients that I had treated at the time of this book's publication.

To put this into clear perspective, think of the situation this way: only two out of 100 advanced-stage cancer patients survive when treated by conventional cancer doctors. In sharp contrast, at least 67 out of every 100 similar people survive when I treat them. There are several reasons:

Unique tests: My clinic offers chemosensitivity tests that determine which types of chemo will most effectively treat a specific individual, while also identifying which drugs, hormones and natural supplements work best for the patient.

Effective process: Before treatment begins, I meet with each patient to develop an effective treatment process based largely on results of the chemosensitivity tests.

Natural treatments: My clinic uses effective and safe natural treatments that not only refrain from damaging the body, while killing cancer and fortifying their natural immunity. These are unlike dangerous drugs used by mainstream oncologists who often administer harmful synthetic substances that often damage patient health and may lead to death.

Cancer obliterated: In most cases my unique treatments generate a 90-plus-percent kill rate of the cancers within such patients. This often enables the patients' immune systems to assume and to successfully carry out the job of completing our fight against the disease, leading to remission. The natural ability of my patients to kill off all remaining cancer increases significantly when I administer superior, effective immune-boosting natural substances.

The 67-percent cancer survival rate generated by Century Wellness Clinic reflects patients who remain alive five years after treatment. Numerous survivors at that point have at least some cancer; among many of these individuals the disease is considered "manageable." Most doctors generally refer to such patients as "cured," particularly individuals who remain in remission after five years.

Consider Me Unique

My treatments sharply boost the possibility of a cure, thanks to the fact that the chemosensitivity tests specify which drugs would work best, and which would be ineffective for each specific patient.

As noted in my newsletters for patients, thanks to the chemosensitivity tests made possible by genomics research, "no other oncologist in the United States can offer this kind of information to his or her patients. What conventional oncologists offer only is what has been the best results of the latest clinical study."

Those reports, which have nothing to do with chemosensitivity tests fail to generate 100-percent accuracy. In fact, many studies embraced by mainstream oncologists are only 30 percent to 50 percent accurate in predicting outcome.

Results show that conventional chemotherapy treatments administered by mainstream oncologists would never help one half to two thirds of Stage IV cancer patients.

Sadly, these patients are merely being poisoned when given chemotherapy, which does little to eliminate cancer--while intensifying their suffering.

Consider Me A Maverick Doctor

Before initially visiting my clinic, many patients soon realize that I'm one of just a handful of working "integrative medical oncologists" worldwide.

This means that I'm fully licensed to practice medicine as a mainstream medical oncologist, while simultaneously working as a board-certified Homeopathic physician using natural treatments.

"I essentially use what some people call 'the best of both medical worlds," I sometimes tell patients. "If I'm giving you the wrong drug, I'm killing you. But that's what traditional oncologists are doing every day."

My unique Century Wellness Clinic, located in Reno, Nevada, in the western United States, fights cancer with harmless and effective natural substances. We do this without the excessive use of the poisonous, dangerous and expensive drugs such as high-dose chemo administered by mainstream oncologists.

Instead, depending on each patient's specific needs and results of the person's chemosensitivity tests, I develop individualized treatment regimens. These often include extremely limited regimens of low-dose chemo along with various natural remedies.

Sadly, mainstream oncologists are forced by the standard medical industry's required protocol to administer deadly regimens of high-dose chemo to all advanced Stage IV cancer patients--with no exceptions.

From the view of many mainstream doctors, I'm threatening to "overturn the proverbial apple cart."

Under such a scenario, would the resulting "public outcry" generate an ideal situation where frustrated patients worldwide and vote-hungry politicians insist that every mainstream oncologist order chemosensitivity tests for all cancer patients?

Patients Yearn for Effective Natural Remedies

Every week, many patients from around the world travel to

Century Wellness Clinic for treatment of cancer or other ailments.

Every week out-of-state license plates are seen in my clinic's parking lot, after patients drive from as far away as Maine, Florida, Alaska, Canada and Mexico.

This influx of visitors provides a consistent and significant boost to the Reno-area economy, generating thousands of hotel room occupancy, with average patient stays at three to four weeks.

A noticeable portion of these patients from every continent except Antarctica. courageously visit my clinic, after being told by mainstream oncologists elsewhere tell to get their affairs in order.

"Never take the word of any doctor who would tell you something like that," I say to patients. "Every patient needs to remain hopeful for as long as possible."

Genetics Research Makes this Possible

Much of Century Wellness Clinic's success in effectively treating cancer patients has been made possible by genomics research, along with my previously mentioned natural remedies.

These technological advances stem from studies inspired by the Human Genome Project, when scientists mapped out the entire human genome from 1990 to 2003.

Findings made possible by genomic research since then have enabled scientists to develop the amazing chemosensitivity tests. I consider this as an essential, vital and necessary tool for cancer doctors when developing effective individual treatment regimens. Yet keep in mind that as previously mentioned, mainstream oncologists insist on ignoring these techniques.

So, as you might imagine, I've been called a "maverick doctor," largely due to my unwillingness to follow the proverbial dictates of allopathic physicians.

You see, I refrain from "following the proverbial pack" of mainstream doctors. Instead, I choose to essentially stand in my own field while proudly enabling my patients to benefit from effective new genomic technologies that other doctors ignore.

Patients Benefit From Choices

My Stage IV cancer patients at Century Wellness Clinic are given a choice regarding their own treatment regimens.

This serves as a sharp contrast from the process offered by mainstream oncologists; those physicians refuse to enable patients to make such decisions.

At my clinic, patients who wish to go conventional at least know about the best drugs for them. At that point, they then have the right answer.

We also send all patients home with the appropriate supplements deemed highly effective for their individual cancers, renewing these products on an as-needed monthly basis.

Chemosensitivity Testing Works Wonders

Every year, tens of thousands of cancer patients in the United States fail to receive genomics-generated cancer chemosensitivity tests that could save their lives.

In countless instances such procedures could prevent certain patients from receiving poisonous chemo that never would help them. When that happens high-dose chemo ravages their bodies. This invariably leads to extremely painful, horrendous and lingering death. Their bodies literally waste away.

"On a widespread social scale, this is a tragedy seemingly beyond belief," I tell patients who inquire about the issue. "The sad fact is that most mainstream oncologists either refuse to or fail to inform their patients that chemosensitivity tests exist."

From the standpoint of the vast majority of allopathic cancer doctors, everything essentially comes down to "guesswork" because of the dismal fact that they refrain from seeking such procedures.

Compounding the problem, as mentioned earlier, medical industry standards require mainstream oncologists to follow "protocol." These puzzling rules mandate that all patients with certain types of advanced-stage cancers always be given specific types of chemo drugs at a pre-designated, high-level; these are administered on pre-set schedules.

Disturbing Results Emerged

By my estimates, in the United States every day nationwide more than 1,300 cancer patients needlessly die such deaths--the equivalent of several jumbo jets crashing into the ocean.

The amount of human suffering is immeasurable on a grand scale.

Yet why do mainstream doctors refuse to recommend such tests? Does mainstream medicine's close ties with Big Pharma--the giant multi-billion-dollar pharmaceutical industry--have anything to do with such the disturbing behavior of these physicians on a grand scale?

While no one can accurately give an irrefutable answer to these critical questions, at least something is clear--patients need to be proactive.

Demand Such Tests

Any person suffering from cancer, particularly advanced Stage IV levels of the disease, should demand the option of taking such tests before any chemo begins. Here are the steps such patients should take:

Access: Before treatment begins, tell the doctor that you want a "cancer chemosensitivity test."

Options: Inquire about what options are available from the doctor for receiving such tests.

History: Ask if the doctor has ever given patients access to such procedures.

Red Flags: Be on the lookout for a "red-flag warning" that if the physician refuses to offer these tests.

Avoid Conventional Oncologists

When I tell my clinic's cancer patients about this, they immediately start avoiding mainstream oncologists--often telling many people that they know to do the same.

I have been issuing such warnings for many years.

In fact, as I noted in my clinic's October 2010 newsletter, "gene testing has the answers" for cancer patients seeking to benefit from cutting-edge technology.

From my view now in my fifth decade of practicing cancer medicine, the development of such tests emerged as "the biggest C-change in all my years of practice with more than 200,000 patient visits."

Patients Appreciate Access

At Century Wellness Clinic, the advent of cancer chemosensitivity testing has made a major difference in the lives of our patients' success levels and improved overall survival rates. These statistics became evident in our present, ongoing five-year, 800-patient study.

Drawing whole blood at my clinic, cancer chemosensitivity tests are relatively simple, easy and productive procedures. Upon their initial visits to Century Wellness, some people with cancer are what homeopaths call "virginal treatment patients."

The designation signifies that those individuals have not yet been treated for their cancers, and therefore have never been subjected to potentially dangerous or deadly treatments such as multiple drugs, radiation, or even major surgery.

For the most part upon their initial visits to Century Wellness, these patients know that their disease is advancing, and their prognosis is guarded. They know their time factors are limited and they want real answers, along with effective non-toxic treatment.

Avoid the Guessing Game

Most of them highly educated and extremely inquisitive, these patients want to avoid getting ensnared in the type of "guessing game" used by mainstream oncologists.

With equal importance, as I clearly stated in my 2010 newsletter, these patients "don't want an oncologist that picks out drugs and throws them against a wall to see if any stick in terms of their own cancer response rates."

A highly trained and experienced member of my professional staff begins the chemosensitivity testing process by taking a patient's whole blood--a very simple and easy procedure. The blood is then handled very carefully, while undergoing stringent packaging and shipping requirements; samples remain good for 96 hours prior the time when the Greek laboratory analyzes the sample.

My personnel always draw the blood on the first part of the week, ensuring that the sample gets to its destination in a safe, preserved and fresh manner.

Upon arrival at the testing laboratory, scientists and lab technicians subject the blood to high-tech tests. At last count, my clinic estimated that at least three labs provide this service--one in Germany, one in Greece and one in South Korea.

We Fine-Tuned Efforts

Following several years of testing, at Century Wellness we found that the Greek Test offers the most important information in terms of the number of chemotherapy agents and supplements that are tested along with the greatest accuracy.

To its credit, the Greek company, RGCC, Research Genetic Cancer Centre, tests at least 12 families of chemotherapy agents and 60 types of supplements.

Once RGCC receives the blood, the testing process takes from 10 days to two weeks for completion of the analysis. To do this, the lab's technicians and scientists sample and harvest the cancer cells--which are then cultured en vitro for gene analysis.

These specific characteristics within the patient's genes are then compared in relationship with how--if at all--the various chemotherapy agents interact with these markers. This way lab technicians determine which of the 12 specific drugs families and 60 supplements work best, if any. In "hormone-driven" cancers the test identifies the best agents for effectively blocking hormonal action.

Upon completing this thorough analysis the Greek laboratory sends results to me. Then, after carefully reviewing this vital data, I construct a protocol involving a unique effective formula that marries the two most effective conventional drugs with all the best supplements. Once a patient agrees to pursue such a strategy, I often combine natural remedies and low-dose chemo to "work smart, rather than merely working hard."

Mainstream Oncologists Destroy the Body

The vast majority of advanced Stage IV cancer patients who visit conventional clinics are merely being poisoned by chemo that fails to do anything to eliminate their cancer. High-dose chemo often causes:

Chemo-brain syndrome: Commonly called "post-chemotherapy cognitive impairment," this hampers or wrecks the patient's cognitive abilities. According to the "Journal of Clinical Oncology," from 20 percent to 30 percent of people who undergo chemotherapy experience at least some form of chemo-brain syndrome. These outcomes have been so disturbing that the Journal of the National Cancer Institute has designated the condition as a real, measurable side effect. Some cancer survivors complain of a degradation of their cognitive abilities, plus decreases in their fluency and memory.

Cardiac toxicities: Sometimes called "cardiotoxicity," this condition occurs when the heart muscle sustains damage or the organ's ejection fraction reduces. These adverse characteristics, in turn, weaken the heart--which fails to adequately pump. The blood circulates with less efficiency than the organ had previously managed to accomplish consistently prior to the chemotherapy treatments. This can be measured by testing the ejection fraction (EF), which should be above 55 percent.

Peripheral neuropathies: This dreaded condition occurs when the body's sensory nerves become damaged or diseased. The numerous adverse symptoms that vary among patients can include the impairment of peripheral nerve organs, plus a hampered ability of movement and a decrease or loss of sensation. A vast array of additional nerve-related damage sometimes occurs, depending on which portion of the body's nerves are effected.

Bone marrow suppression: Sometimes called "myelotoxicity," this adverse medical condition generates one or all of numerous highly adverse effects. Besides the potential loss of normal blood clotting, some patients experience a severe infections that result from a decrease in the white cells responsible for providing immunity. Just as destructive, another condition called "anemia" can severely hamper the essential life-giving ability of red blood cells to carry oxygen.

Generalized rashes: Often lasting from five to 20 days, or perhaps much longer, this condition can generate bothersome itchiness, bumps, cracked or blistered skin, debilitating pain, and a variety of other adverse conditions such as secondary infections due to cracks or blisters.

Death: Conventional oncologists typically prefer to avoid discussing this topic at length with patients, but there is no escaping the fact that the needless or reckless over-use of chemotherapy often results in unnecessary death. Quite predictably many patients suffer from some or even all of the previously mentioned symptoms triggered by chemo, before dying from severe levels of these adverse side effects. Most allopathic cancer doctors refrain from admitting this disturbing fact--many of their patients are killed by the highly toxic and poisonous chemo, rather than succumbing to the cancer itself.

Better Choices Available

As a licensed oncologist I'm required by law and by industry protocol to give each Stage IV cancer patient the option of having conventional high-dose chemo "treatments"--instances where such a strategy would be required of standard oncologists.

The vast majority of people with advanced-stage cancer who visit my clinic freely choose to avoid high doses of dangerous drugs. These patients usually follow my recommendation of a low-dose insulin potentiated chemo regimen, coupled with effective natural remedies--as determined by genetic testing.

For these individuals, my clinic administers low-dose fractionated insulin-potentiated regimens often referred to as "IPT." This technique "tricks the cancers" into opening up certain biological receptors. This happens due to a cancer's enhanced supply of insulin receptors.

These attributes leave the cancer open to potentially effective attacks by apoptosis-producing natural Poly-MVA administered by my clinic's medical personnel. This tactic often works because cancers can only thrive on simple sugars.

As a result, the cancers often die or go into remission, robbing the disease of its ultimate goal of killing the patient.

Important Book Emerged

One of my many patients became so impressed with this process that she wrote a compelling book about her positive experience being treated at Century Wellness Clinic.

Las Vegas-based businesswoman Diana Warren chronicled her story in "Say No to Radiation and Conventional Chemo--Winning My Battle Against Stage II Breast Cancer."

Prior to visiting my office Warren had gone to numerous

mainstream oncologists. All of those medical professionals had insisted that she endure high-dose chemo treatments and radiation therapy.

Brave, intelligent and charismatic, Warren refused to cave in to their dangerous medical procedures. Instead, she let common sense serve as her guide, while ignoring the reckless protocol of mainstream physicians.

Warren undertook an in-depth research regimen, eventually deciding to visit my Reno-based clinic 450 miles from Las Vegas. Then, at my urging, Warren decided to take the "Greek Test," the chemosensitivity analysis.

The test results arrived within several weeks. Right away I worked with Warren in developing her personalized treatment regimen. We used a combination of the medications and supplements that the analysis had identified as the most effective for her body and particular type of cancer.

Warren's unique and specialized low-dose chemo treatment regimen began within several weeks at Century Wellness Clinic. Her cancer went into remission soon afterward, and at the time of this book's publication she had remained in remission for more than four years.

Numerous Positive Outcomes

Although I would never refer to myself in such glowing terms, numerous doctors and industry observers refer to me as a "virtual rock star within the medical industry."

Rooms filled with Homeopaths and their assistants often erupt into applause or give standing ovations as soon as I enter some medical industry conferences.

Always in high demand to attend such functions, I usually visit from six to 10 medical industry seminars yearly throughout the United States. You see, I continually learn more about fighting cancer while always developing effective, natural ways to fight the disease.

The positive focus on me and my clinic's techniques intensified when an intelligent and highly respected celebrity, Suzanne Somers, mentioned these critical details in worldwide media forums. Somers became so impressed that she described my clinic's cancer treatment procedures in her runaway 2010 bestseller, "Knockout: Interviews With Doctors Who are Curing Cancer--And How to Prevent Getting It in the First Place."

Huge percentages of my patients learn of Century Wellness Clinic via positive word-of-mouth from other people previously treated at my clinic. Streams of my patients first learn about me in Somers' book, or from the many books that I have written, or co-authored, or from publications where other writers praise my medical procedures.

Groundbreaking Doctor Pushes the Proverbial Envelope

An internationally acclaimed Los Angeles physician and surgeon, Doctor Patrick Soon-Shiong, has generally been using the same overall type of genomic-related testing and cancer treatment that my Century Wellness Clinic has been using with much success.

With an estimated personal worth of $11 billion, Soon-Shiong has been called "a genius, a showman, an innovator and a hypster," CBS News correspondent Doctor Sanjay Gupta, said in a "60 Minutes" program segment first aired on Dec. 7, 2014.

Like me, Soon-Shiong has had his advance-stage cancer treatment methodology come into question from some mainstream doctors. Those physicians insist that more time is needed to determine if such genomic testing and IPT treatments are effective and worthy of being recommended.

Yet as if echoing statements that I have made for more than 10 years, Soon-Shiong told Gupta that patients suffering from advance-stage cancer lack the luxury of time needed to wait for extensive testing and federal approval of new treatments.

"I'm incredibly encouraged to say that we are on the path,"

Soon-Shiong told "60 Minutes." "And the technology to do these things is not just hypothetical."

Soon-Shiong insists that scientists are learning to unmask cancer's molecular secrets, thanks largely to advances in DNA technology, coupled with a high-speed genome sequencing machine that he developed.

Similar to a process that I implemented at my clinic, the billionaire doctor prefers to have his advance-stage cancer patients undergo genomic testing. Like me, he strives to determine which specific drugs have the greatest probability of effectively killing the cancer of each patient.

Another similarity to my clinic's general protocol emerges from the fact that Soon-Shiong prefers administering low-dose chemo treatments.

Similar Overall Techniques Generate Success

In yet another significant similarity, Soon-Shiong insists that many people have a mistaken belief that cancer cells merely "grow." Instead, because of a mysterious and still-understood genetic mutation, the worst cancers essentially have *the inability to die*.

In our separate, unaffiliated medical practices while still employing similar overall strategies, Soon-Shiong's clinic and mine share a mutual professional and highly focused obsession with using genomic technology to determine the characteristics of cancer's strange mutation.

Ultimately, this often results in an improved long-term survival rate, always starting with a thorough analysis of each individual patient's genomic structure and specific type of cancer.

In best-case scenarios, these advances in cancer diagnosis and treatment ultimately lead to instances where the disease becomes categorized as completely gone or when cancer evolves into a "chronic health conditions" rather than fatal.

"Overall, these advancements are clicking into gear at a far greater pace than many people realize," I sometimes tell patients. "The old way of treating cancer patients with high-dose chemo should quickly emerge as 'a thing of the past,' replaced by a much more effective era."

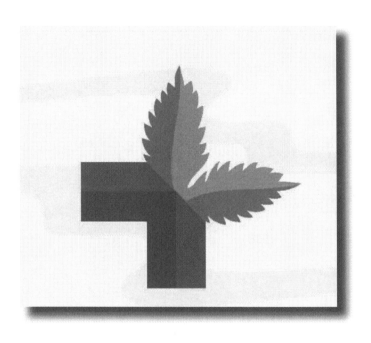

Century Wellness Clinic Leads the Way

Almost every day the whole world seems to be banging on my clinic's door, eager and desperate to benefit from substantial advances in genomic technology.

Yet amazingly only an infinitesimal fraction of the 7 billion living people worldwide knows that my clinic uses these amazing anti-cancer techniques.

My office doors are always open weekdays, except on a handful of U.S. holidays and during the brief span from Christmas through New Year's Day.

As you might very well imagine, my office phones are continually "ringing off the hook" while people ask for appointments.

Many patients tell me that they're pleased and delighted upon discovering that my staff is eager to answer any questions that they might have.

Demand Continues to Intensify

The patient load at Century Wellness Clinic continues on a steady increase. Every step of the way we strive to make the process as stress-free and easy as possible for each person eager for an examination and treatment.

I' have already stated the following in the first chapter, but I need to re-emphasize the details here because the important facts are essential to all my patients:

Many people visiting for the first time admit they're impressed by the fact that nearly two-thirds of my Stage IV cancer patients remain alive and in remission from the disease--4.5 years after their initial treatments at Century Wellness Clinic.

Remember, this means that six out of every 10 worst-stage cancer patients that I treat remain alive, most relatively healthy and capable of enjoying life to the fullest.

By contrast, according to numerous nationwide medical reports, only two out of every 100 Stage IV cancer patients survive when treated by mainstream oncologists.

So, knowing these details, who would you choose--the doctors required to administer high-dose poison in all such cases, or me, an expert at administering an effective combination of low-dose chemo, natural remedies and healthy supplements?

Take These Important Steps

To help optimize results and make their excursions as stress-free as possible, all first-time patients visiting Century Wellness Clinic can:

Call: 775-827-0707, or toll free 877-789-0707; tell the receptionist your health situation, so that we can start the process of potentially making a reservation.

Records: Upon making a reservation, you must bring copies of your records from your current doctor, or send us that information before arriving. This information should include any and all available reports regarding oncology, pathology, surgery, chemotherapy, X-rays, scans, laboratory tests, narrative summaries, and a list of all medications and supplements.

Frailty: Like all doctors, we generally are unable to treat patients who have become "extremely frail;" under this condition the person's body mass and weight have dropped to precipitously low levels--while muscles have nearly disappeared.

Prior Treatments: Preferably before their first visit to Century Wellness, patients should avoid being treated elsewhere by mainstream oncologists. The high-dose chemo and radiation administered by those doctors seriously weakens and damages the body--thereby decreasing the potential effectiveness of subsequent treatments. Homeopaths refer to people with cancer who refrain from chemo and radiation prior to visiting doctors of natural medicine as "virginal treatment patients." Although we prefer treating "virginal patients," in many instances my clinic accepts people with cancer who already have been treated by conventional oncologists. In order to be accepted, such candidates must communicate with a member of my staff before a decision is made.

Travel & Accommodations: New and returning patients make their own arrangements for travel and lodging. The Reno area has numerous high-quality hotels and restaurants at mid-range and high-end prices. Car rentals via Reno-Tahoe International Airport are available for those who travel by air, and shuttle services are provided by most major hotel-casinos in the region.

Location: Century Wellness Clinic is at 521 Hammill Lane in South Reno, an ideal site just one block from on-ramps and off-ramps to U.S. Interstate 580--one of the region's two primary highways. A north-south arterial, I-580 provides easy access to the airport, all of the region's primary hotels, and the region's primary east-west highway, U.S. Interstate 80. Travel time to or from the airport and the clinic is about 10 minutes.

Activities: During "free" time when not undergoing medical examinations or treatments, patients, their relatives or friends have a vast array of options for fun, relaxing, energizing or restful activities. The high-desert region surrounding Reno, which is at 4,500 feet above sea level, has hundreds of miles of hiking trails providing panoramic views. The city is just a one-hour drive from Lake Tahoe, an ideal summer playground. Nestled in the Sierra at 6,200 feet above sea level, as North America's largest alpine lake, Tahoe has easy access to dozens of ski resorts popular during winter. Just as enticing, the historic Comstock Lode mining town of Virginia City, where the legendary writer Mark Twain began his journalism career for the "Territorial Enterprise" in the 1860s, is just a 30-minute drive southeast of Reno. Virginia City has numerous popular attractions including museums, and historic saloons such as the the world famous Bucket of Blood saloon.

Expected stays: Patients visiting for initial examinations and chemosensitivity testing usually stay from several days to one week. Those undergoing treatment regimens of low-dose chemo, effective natural remedies and supplements usually stay from two to three weeks. Subsequent visits for standard examinations are usually recommended for patients who have undergone treatments, so that I can monitor each person's progress in beating cancer. Follow-up visits for examinations usually are arranged in three- or six-month, or one-year intervals; these spans hinge on the type of cancer a patient had, the current suspected severity of the disease; and whether the cancer has gone into--or seems to progressing into--remission.

Additional treatment: Some patients occasionally require or request follow-up treatment regimens if their cancer remains active following the initial round.

Various ailments: Century Wellness Clinic treats patients suffering from many types of ailments, particularly cancer. We treat all types of the disease in any bodily area and at every level of severity; besides advanced Stage IV cancer, the clinic treats patients suffering from less severe levels including Stage II and Stage III. Patients need to know that unless effectively treated all types of cancer can worsen to the dreaded Stage IV; the worst-stage cancers invariably lead to death unless successfully treated. In addition, many patients learn prior to their initial visits to Century Wellness that mainstream oncologists strive to administer poisonous and deadly high-dose chemo to patients suffering from the less severe Stage II or Stage III levels of the disease--not just Stage IV.

Critical Patient Choices

Keep in mind that as previously stated, throughout every phase of each patient's examinations and treatment I give the patient the option of making critical choices.

This marks a sharp contrast from the style of mainstream oncologists, who essentially say without using such specific words: "It's my way, or the highway."

I give each patient the option of receiving natural remedies that are proven highly effective, always with the patient's physical and mental well-being in mind.

In doing so, I'm essentially following the philosophy of Doctor Benjamin Rush, a signer of the Declaration of Independence and the personal physician of U.S. President George Washington.

"Unless we put medical freedom into the Constitution, the time will come when medicine will organize into an undercover dictatorship," said Rush, a founding father of the United States who died in 1813 at age 67. "To restrict the art of healing to one class of men and deny equal privileges to others will cause a Bastille of medical science.

"All such laws are un-American and despotic, and have no place in a republic. The Constitution of this republic should make a special privilege for medical freedom."

To the detriment of all types of patients, no such provisions were included in the USA's founding documents. Since then mainstream doctors have run roughshod over patients' rights; these physicians have used their political allies to implement and control federal agencies that require or sanction the use of ineffective, costly, and poisonous deadly drugs.

Whole Body and Soul

Effectively treating patients can only happen when addressing the whole body, the mind and what I sometimes call the person's "positive spirit or soul."

Unlike mainstream oncologists who poison the entire body in an effort "to fix an isolated cancer," I incorporate a whole-body strategy using mostly natural remedies.

Besides administering low-dose chemo with natural

remedies, personnel at my clinic also help address numerous issues in order to improve each patient's overall health. Among these critical health-enhancing tactics that mainstream oncologists ignore are:

Balance: We show each patient how to achieve a balanced lifestyle using an ideal combination of rest, exercise, sleep, nutrition and activities suited for emotional harmony.

Detoxify: Clean the body of foreign or unnatural substances that are likely to damage overall health, while sometimes also sometimes triggering cancer.

Diet: The common saying that "you are what you eat" remains true, sometimes leading to cancer due to unhealthy diets. So, we teach patients about good nutrition.

Empower: As previously stated, we give each patient choices about treatment, recovery and strategies to achieve or to maintain optimal health.

Information: We teach patients the critical details that they must know to detect, prevent and control cancer.

Sugar: We teach each patient that common sugars, particular when ingested in high amounts, are a leading cause of cancer--which "love and thrives" on this substance.

Supplements: Use the supplements identified by chemosensitivity testing as the most helpful for a specific cancer patient; these products contain vitamins, minerals and various herbs. They serve as the backbone for good overall physical, mental and spiritual health.

Target Specific Cancers

I have developed unique, individualized strategies to effectively battle each form of cancer.

This is unlike mainstream oncologists who--as previously stated--use an ill-advised and ineffective "one-size-fits-all" approach to almost every form of the disease.

By analyzing an individual's chemosensitivity test,

physical examination and medical records, I'm able to marry the best natural remedies in combination with low-dose chemo, along with supplements identified as the most effective for the person.

Doctors classify each form of cancer based on the bodily area where the disease started. Compounding the challenge, each type of cancer has a unique growth rate, pattern of spreading and response to specific treatments.

Many physicians and particularly Homeopaths have deemed me as perhaps the world's premiere expert at developing and matching the ideal and most effective treatment for each type of cancer.

Chemosensitivity tests are particularly helpful because each person has a unique, one-of-a-kind genomic structure unlike any other person.

Risk Factors Play a Role

Intense and continuous worldwide genomic research has been identifying and confirming what many physicians have suspected for a long time.

Genomic research has confirmed that some individuals have a greater likelihood than the general population of developing specific types of cancer.

For instance, women from some families have a far greater chance of developing breast cancer than most females throughout the general population.

At least some good news has emerged. Scientists have confirmed that the inherited probability of cancer is less prevalent than previously thought.

As a result, some researchers and medical facilities have informally categorized most cancer causes as instances where the individual is a victim of "bad luck."

Many severe risk factors sharply increase the probability of getting cancer. Besides smoking or chewing tobacco, these include exposure to chemicals, ultraviolet light, free radicals in foods, red or processed meats, sugar, air pollution and many more.

In addition, each specific risk factor increases a person's chances of getting certain cancers. For instance, smoking or chewing tobacco sharply increases a person's risk of developing cancers of the lung, tongue, mouth, larynx, and other organs. Scientists blame most skin cancers on excessive exposure to the sun or suntanning machines.

Most tumors are benign or lacking cancer; such tumors are usually non-threatening, except in rare exceptions.

In all instances of cancer, a person's chances of "being cured" increase drastically the sooner the disease is discovered and treated; cancers that are allowed to grow and spread over extended periods without being treated sharply increase the chances of developing into deadly advanced Stage IV levels of the disease.

My "War Plan" in Fighting Cancer

In the fight against cancer, patients at Century Wellness Clinic might think of me as a proverbial five-star general or a commander-in-chief.

Under my continual command the clinic's staff administers at least 17 strategies, many that I have personally designed to destroy cancer. With added importance, some of these strategies strive to put each patient on a pathway toward optimal overall health.

Besides the unique chemosensitivity testing of whole blood, one of these key techniques briefly mentioned earlier involves the low-dose fractionated regimens sometimes called "IPT."

As previously stated, when using a unique system that I personally developed, the process strives to "trick" or "fool" the disease into opening certain receptors within the cancer's cells. This happens in part because cancers desperately crave energy-producing sugar and oxygen.

I work to ensure that this natural process opens biological receptors. When this happens the cancer is left wide-open to horrific attacks, while the rest of the body remains unharmed and safe.

The typical weaponry that I employ here involves a natural substance, the harmless and effective Poly-MVA expertly administered by my staff. This is usually done on alternate days with low-dose fractionated chemotherapy, levels much smaller and far less harmful to the body than chemo typically administered by mainstream oncologists.

Napoleonic Battles Against Cancer

Although despotic, often cruel and heartless, the famed French Emperor and General Napoléon Bonaparte of the early 19th Century remains world-famous for his dastardly war tactics of suddenly attacking enemies using extreme unconventional tactics.

At least within the realm of battling cancer, many of my patients think of me as using "Napoleonic battle plans against the disease within the practices of both oncology and Homeopathy."

Highly detailed books could be separately written and published about each of my most popular and effective cancer-fighting strategies. Besides chemosensitivity tests, IPT, and low-dose fractionated chemotherapy, here is a brief summary of some of the most effective methods frequently used at Century Wellness Clinic:

Healthful water: Because healthful, pure water can boost energy while ridding the body of harmful and potentially cancerous impurities, we provide patients with access to pH 9.0 "alkaline H2O pH therapy." The water is at an optimal alkaline level, the opposite from the harmful acidic range. This strategy serves an important role because cancer thrives within an acidic environment; the pH levels of most cancer patients are typically far more acidic than alkaline.

Nutritional guidance: What a person chooses to eat plays a critical role in either generating or preventing cancer. Many of these "poor" and "good" choices hinge on whether a particular food is within the healthful alkaline or unhealthy acidic ranges. We show patients meal plans developed for their unique personal situations. These details can be found in my hot-selling book, the "Forsythe Anti-Cancer Diet;" it's available in paper or e-reader form via all major bookstores and online eBook venues.

Individualized nutrition: Besides the advice on diet briefly mentioned above, we develop cancer-fighting and cancer-preventing regimens that include specific foods, vitamins, and herbs. As I often tell patients, natural substances such as these generally are far more preferable than unnatural or synthetic drugs typically administered by mainstream oncologists. Besides helping to boost overall health, such products serve as just one of the many ways that we help give the body a fighting, natural chance against cancer.

Immune Enhancement: Cancer typically compromises or weakens the body's immune system, often robbing the person of energy and the ability to fight the disease. To counteract this detrimental condition, we administer a Vitamin-C high-dose immune booster that patients receive intravenously as a standard procedure. Often loaded with vital additional vitamins and supplements, these immune-enhancing sessions often sharply increase the body's natural ability to battle certain ailments--particularly cancer. Besides cancer patients, my clinic treats people with other health issues that compromise or weaken immunity.

Biological Response Modifiers: Besides the immune enhancement technique listed immediately above, we also employ "biological response modifiers" that are sometimes called "BRMs." Remember that as mentioned earlier, the effective strategies that I employ typically strive to kill at least 90 percent of a patient's cancer, and from that point the person's immune system plays a critical role in fighting and successfully killing the remainder of the disease. Similar to substances naturally produced by the body and often created by scientists in laboratories, BRMs super-charge the body's natural response to infection and to cancer. This "immunotherapy" treatment process enhances the body's immune systems, particularly natural defenses against cancer. Also, because my clinic serves patients with ailments other than cancer, we sometimes use BRMs to affectively address such adverse conditions as rheumatoid arthritis. Although comprised of natural substances, the administering of BRMs on extremely rare occasion generates adverse symptoms such as diarrhea, nausea, vomiting and loss of appetite. Thus, BRMs should only be taken in a professional medical environment that monitors patients.

Bio-Oxidative Therapy: A super-powerful tool among natural healing methods, the natural process called "bio-oxidative therapy" serves as a stong anti-oxidant and cancer killer. One of only a small percentage of physicians to use this strategy, I have learned first-hand many times that bio-oxidative therapy robs cancer of low oxygen that the disease needs to live, grow and thrive. Unlike humans and all mammals, cancer gets its oxygen from the fermentation process, rather than breathing from the environment. At my recommendation and upon patient approval, I use bio-oxidative therapy to surround cancer cells with oxygen. This high-oxygen environment can significantly decrease the disease's ability to grow and to divide. Meantime, this therapy typically stimulates receptors in white blood cells, thus boosting the immune system and fortifying the body's natural strength and effectiveness in attacking cancer. Perhaps just as impressive, this therapy increases the body's natural production of interferon, interleukin-2 and tumor necrosis factor--all factors that sharply boost the body's natural cancer fighting processes. Meantime, bio-oxidative therapy also often improves the health of patients who have been ill, thanks to the ability of this process to increase oxygen tension in bodily tissues.

Lifestyle guidance: Clinic staff members often teach or suggest ways for an individual patient to enjoy life to the fullest extent possible. Such positive behavioral changes often make the person feel better both physically and emotionally, thereby decreasing the likelihood that a cancer will worsen or return. When giving this advice, my personnel consider numerous simultaneous factors including the person's type and severity of cancer, level of remission, overall health, and all other ailments currently experienced by the individual.

Professional referrals: As a highly experienced doctor with extensive medical industry contacts throughout Northern Nevada and worldwide, I sometimes refer patients who need additional services to other medical professionals ranging from surgeons to radiologists.

Second opinions: After initially receiving the diagnosis of physicians elsewhere, some people visit Century Wellness Clinic to seek a "second opinion" from me or other doctors on my staff. Sometimes we reach similar conclusions, although in numerous instances either I or my personnel generate findings that differ from what the patient had been told elsewhere.

Coping skills: Century Wellness Clinic offers individual and group counseling, unlike the vast majority of mainstream oncologists and cancer treatment facilities nationwide. At my clinic, skilled advisers highly knowledgeable in medicine and optimal lifestyles teach patients or their families how to cope and excel in key issues. Patients and their families learn optimal ways to administer effective healthcare, plus suggested methods on handling daily lifestyle tasks or personal responsibilities.

Patients Deserve Priority Status

At Century Wellness Clinic, every patient gets "priority status;" they all deserve and receive respect without being ignored or told, "Do this and do that. Take this poison, because you have no other choice."

The doctors and personnel at my facility strongly embrace this highly coveted mission statement. We strive to show each patient that the clinic truly cares, while effectively working in an effort to achieve the best possible results.

Blessed with a keen knowledge of the art and science of medicine, I continually draw upon all treatment modalities ranging from the most advanced conventional therapies to mainstream medicine. All along, I also incorporate the most effective remedies of Homeopathic medicine, primarily natural therapies ignored by mainstream oncologists.

Using these medical systems as a solid foundation for giving all patients the best possible care, I have developed four options uniquely designed to fulfill their desires:

One: Fractionated conventional chemotherapy alone

Two: Fractional chemotherapy, plus Homeopathic treatments including Insulin Potentiated Therapy (IPT) Lite (TM).

Three: Complimentary Homeopathic and/or naturopathic modalities alone

Four: Best supportive therapy

Based on my intensive studies, I have discovered that superior results occur when using combination treatments of: IPT with fractionated (low-dose) chemotherapy; Homeopathic intravenous remedies; and immune-stimulating supplements including organic herbs.

Along with my staff throughout the course of treating thousands of patients, I have developed intense studies on: Paw-Paw, a naturally grown substance deemed highly effective in cancer treatment; Poly-MVA, a uniquely formulated combination of minerals and amino acids designed to support cellular energy and promote overall good health, while also highly effective for treating cancer; the Forsythe Immune Protocol, a highly effective immune-enhancing process that I personally developed to

313

significantly boost positive results in the treatment of my cancer patients; and a combination of the Forsythe Immune Protocol, CST and IPT--which means chemosensitivity testing, followed by IPT.

A "Bill of Rights" for Patients

Determined to counteract the "dogmatic rules" imposed by mainstream oncologists who refuse to allow patients to make vital choices regarding their own health, I have developed an essential "Bill of Rights" that all people with cancer can embrace. Among some of the most important proclamations:

Positive attitude: Each patient has a right to refrain from becoming afraid or discouraged, always cognizant that at various times in recent years medical literature has chronicled cures for all types of cancer.

Alternative path: Patients have a right to chose a unique, extremely rare integrative medical oncologist such as me because I'm highly skilled at treating their entire bodies with harmless and effective natural remedies--plus drugs when necessary.

High-dose chemo: Patients have a right to refuse extensive high-dose chemo regimens that mainstream oncologists insist on administering. When and if such a refusal is made, the patient should have a right to seek out the services of an extremely rare integrative medical oncologist such as me--capable of administering effective natural remedies.

Remain skeptical: Patients have a right to "keep an open mind about issues," while also remaining skeptical when reading or hearing about the supposed results of various clinical studies--particularly instances where two or more drugs are used.

Show spunk: Each patient has a right to peacefully "stand his or her own ground" as a self-preservation measure. Such instances might involve politely leaving an oncologist's office when the doctor mentions "hospice care" or "getting your affairs in order." Such statements indicate that the physician has given up on you; all patients have a right to embrace an attitude that: "I will never give up on myself."

Food choices: Patients have a right and a responsibility to themselves to adopt good eating habits, following the advice of their Homeopaths, physicians and dietitians.

Avoid unnecessary tests: Patients have a right to refuse over-testing, particularly procedures that involve radiation; radiological scans that target various areas of the body's overall immune system are particularly dangerous. Such procedures endanger overall health, increasing the likelihood that immune defenses will fail to work at optimal levels.

Alternative medicines: Patients have a right to know about, to use and to benefit from effective natural remedies that mainstream oncologists refuse to mention or to use. Of particular importances are beneficial supplements that often emerge as extremely helpful and essential in fighting cancer; supplements also eliminate carcinogens and toxins from the body.

Beware of media: Patients have a right and a responsibility to themselves to remain wary of advertisements or promotions that strive to fool them. For instance, some cancer centers claim to have the latest "pinpointed radiology procedures."

Refuse certain surgeries: Particularly among those with advanced Stage IV cancer, patients have a right to avoid a doctor's insistence that they undergo aggressive surgical procedures. These include second-look operations and devastating head-and-neck surgeries requiring tracheotomy and/or gastric feeding tubes.

Limit drugs: Patients have a right to limit the amount of drugs that they take. Whenever possible a patient should be able to take the smallest number of drugs, administered at the lowest-possible doses needed to fight their cancer. This strategy can minimize or prevent the destruction of the person's vital immune system.

Patients Praise Me

I receive heart-felt, compelling and emotional letters or emails each week from all over the world, sent by patients extremely grateful for their improved health.

"I'm so grateful to remain alive," is a phrase signifying a common theme. "I'm eternally grateful for the new lease on life that you have given me."

Some of my now-healthy former patients retell their stories, recounting the fact that they had previously been told elsewhere that: "You are going to die."

Imagine being informed that you are definitely going to be killed within a certain limited number of weeks or months, only to subsequently learn after finally being treated by me that you are going to live.

While glad to receive these messages, I refrain from dwelling on them--partly due to the need to continually concentrate on my job of "saving" as many people as possible.

Of course, not all of my patients survive. Yet as previously stated, the five-year survival rate of my advanced Stage IV cancer patients is far greater than the national average. Remember, according to my clinic's current study involving 850 patients, only two out of every 100 Stage IV cancer patients treated by mainstream oncologists survive, while 67 of such people that I treat remain alive at five years.

Essential Details

As previously mentioned, even following my success in treating cancer patients, I never can, have or will issue any guarantee that any patient will be cured or experience a significant improvement in his or her overall medical condition.

With this clearly understood, readers should remain fully cognizant of the fact that the details that I have provided in this book are strictly for educational and informational purposes only.

In addition, you should refrain from considering any or all

statements that I have made here as medical advice--specifically because at this point we can assume that you are not yet a patient of mine.

I only make specific diagnosis and issue recommendations individually to each of my patients after conducting a thorough physical examination and reviewing medical records.

With these "disclaimer" factors clearly understood, my clinic welcomes inquiries from potential patients. Also, prospective patients should know that Century Wellness Clinic is an out-patient facility without overnight accommodations.

About the Author

James W. Forsythe, M.D., H.M.D., has long been considered one of the most respected physicians in the United States, particularly for his treatment of cancer and the legal use of human growth hormone. In the mid-1960s, Dr. Forsythe graduated with honors from University California at Berkeley and earned his Medical Degree from University of California, San Francisco, before spending two years residency in Pathology at Tripler Army Hospital, Honolulu. After a tour of duty in Vietnam, he returned to San Francisco and completed an internal medicine residency and an oncology fellowship. He is also a world-renowned speaker and author. He has co-authored, been mentioned in and/or written chapters in bestsellers. To name a few: "The Human Genome Playbook for Disrupting Cancer;" "An Alternative Medicine Definitive Guide to Cancer;" "Knockout, Interviews with Doctors who are Curing Cancer" Suzanne Somers' number one bestseller; "The Ultimate Guide To Natural Health, Quick Reference A-Z Directory of Natural Remedies for Diseases and Ailments;" "Anti-Aging Cures;" "The Healing Power of Sleep;" and "Compassionate Oncology ~ What Conventional Cancer Specialists Don't Want You To Know;" and "Obaminable Care," "Complete Pain," "Natural Pain Killers," and "Your Secret to the Fountain of Youth ~ What They Don't Want You to Know About HGH Human Growth Hormone," "Take Control of Your Cancer," "Understanding and Surviving Obamacare," "About Death from a Cancer Doctor's Perspective," "Dr. Forsythe's Whey Protein Anti-Aging Formula," and the "Emergency Radiation Medical Handbook."

Contact Information

Dr. James W. Forsythe, M.D., H.M.D.
Century Wellness Clinic
521 Hammill Lane, Reno, NV 89511-1004
775-827-0707
Website: DrForsythe.com
Email: RenoWellnessDr @ yahoo.com

Addendum

Marijuana's Interaction with Herbs, Supplements and Drugs

As previously mentioned in extensive detail, marijuana can be extremely dangerous when mixed with drugs.

You also need to know that some scientists or practitioners of natural medicine believe that marijuana generates adverse reactions when used with herbs or even generally harmless supplements.

These factors are essential for you to remember, although there supposedly has never been a fatal overdose that involved taking only cannabis--without other drugs.

Obviously, more conclusive study is needed. Also, as previously mentioned, disagreement remains on any apparent or possible dangers that supposedly involve marijuana--either eaten or smoked.

At least from the view of some medical industry practitioners, this same warning should hold true for anyone who mixes cannabis with herbs and supplements.

Amid such controversy, you always should remain cognizant of these potential problems, whether using marijuana for medicinal purposes or recreation.

Become Cautious When Considering these Conclusions

Readers need to be forewarned that many of the anti-marijuana, anti-herb and anti-supplement conclusions described in this section were actually amassed in conjunction with a federal agency that maintains close ties to Big Pharma.

The U.S. federal National Institutes of Health, often known as NIH, maintains long-standing alliances with the world's largest pharmaceutical companies--plus physicians and laboratory personnel closely allied to those firms. From earlier sections of this book, you known that the federal government's various health agencies and the Food and Drug Administration universally make nothing but negative, untrue and irresponsble statements about marijuana (and also natural substances).

Worsening matters, many of these negative and possibly false statements criticizing marijuana when used en tandem with herbs or supplements actually were compiled in conjunction with university medical schools that also have close ties to the pharmaceutical industry.

All along, however, I also have found no solid, irrefutable evidence or reports concluding that the research was conducted in a manner designed to be intentionally biased against marijuana, herbs and supplements.

Also on the plus side, much of this information has been either compiled or distributed by the highly respected "National Standard"--sometimes described by the phrase on its logo, "National Medicine Quality Standard."

As described online, this Massachusets-based international research collaboration "systematically reviews scientific evidence on complimentary and alternative medicine."

The National Standard also has earned a well-deserved solid and positive reputation for its groundbreaking work in providing essential information about herbal medicine and dietary supplements.

Various Reports Deserve Attention

Based on a wide variety of sources, either questionable or reliable, here are some of the many possible dangers or physical reactions when mixing or using marijuana with natural herbs or supplements:

Blood sugar levels: Some medical professionals insist that marijuana lowers blood sugar levels, while others disagree. With this potential problem clearly in mind, consumers might want to consider using extreme caution with marijuana--or avoid that drug altogether--whenever taking herbs or supplements in an effort to lower blood sugar. For people who insist on taking marijuana while also using herbs and supplements to control blood sugar, I recommend continually monitoring blood sugar levels; adjust doses to prevent blood sugars from becoming critically low.

Blood pressure: Marijuana sometimes causes blood pressure to decrease. People using this drug should use caution or avoid taking cannabis when also using supplements and herbs deemed effective at lowering blood pressure.

Bleeding risk: As over-the-top as this might seem, some practitioners of natural medicine believe that using marijuana with natural herbs and substances might increase the risk of bleeding. Once again, such possible dangers remain a matter of dispute. Nonetheless, until much more scientific research is done, I recommend taking a "cautionary approach--just in case." Of primary concern in this regard is Ginkgo biloba, which reportedly has caused bleeding in some people who also were using marijuana. Saw palmetto and garlic are also of concern, but those apparent problems have been reported on a less frequent basis. Once again, although the supposed dangers in such instances are arguable, I recommend taking the precautionary approach of avoiding Ginkgo biloba, garlic and saw palmetto when using marijuana; you can take those natural substances while avoiding the drug.

Liver function: The liver's vital enzyme and chemical processing features reportedly malfunction when simultaneously addressing herbs and supplements along with marijuana. According to at least some reports, the marijuana in such instances interferes with the liver's cytochrome P450 enzyme system. This failure of the liver to perform at optimal levels reportedly sometimes results in excessively high levels of herbs and supplements within the blood. Additionally, such instances might alter the effects of certain herbs and substances.

Sleepiness: Some people reportedly become extremely drowsy when using marijuana with herbs or supplements.

Additional Precautions Become Necessary

A vast array of other clinical reports conclude that marijuana may also adversely interact with anti-depressants, barbiturates and various other Big Pharma drugs. These range from pain relievers and opium-based pharmaceuticals to anti-inflammatory products.

While those conclusions come as no surprise, a somewhat perplexing overall pattern emerges. These findings also characterize marijuana as interacting adversely with herbs and substances used to generate or to treat:

Blood vessel width

Heart disorders

Hormonal issues

Immune system enhancement

Increase appetite

Lung disorders

Nausea and vomiting

Nervous system disorders

Skin disorders

Stomach disorders

The underlying cause of AIDS, a retrovirus infection called HIV

Toxic liver conditions

Big Pharma Viewpoint

As predictable as every sunrise, a Website closely tied to Big Pharma--Drugs.com--lists more than 500 drugs known to interact with marijuana. Remember, Big Pharma continually blasts the effectiveness of cannabis and says nothing positive about the drug, primarily because the substance is a natural plant that cannot be patented.

Thus, eager to obliterate any positive reputation that marijuana might have to some consumers, Big Pharma could quite possibly be listing far too many supposedly negative interactions that marijuana has with specific drugs.

Even so, marijuana obviously has extremely dangerous and

potentially deadly interactions with many of the world's most notorious narcotics and even some "normally harmless" over-the-counter drugs.

Besides aspirin and caffeine, according to Drugs.com, marijuana interacts with such basic mild analgesics as acetaminophen--a common ingredient in popular brand-name over-the-counter painkillers including Tylenol.

For a full listing of the many hundreds of various generic and brand-name drugs that Big Pharma says interact with marijuana, visit Drugs.com